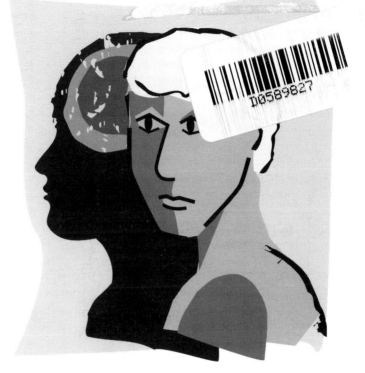

HEAD INJURY

A Practical Guide

Trevor Powell

HEADWAY

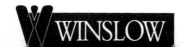

WINSLOW

DEDICATION

FOR MERIEL AND ROSEANNE
Two very special women

First published in 1994 by **Headway National Head Injuries Association Limited**,
7 King Edward Court, King Edward Street, Nottingham NG1 1EW, United Kingdom and
Winslow Press Limited, Telford Road, Bicester, Oxon OX6 0TS, United Kingdom.
Reprinted 1995

02-1717/Printed in the United Kingdom by Hobbs the Printers of Southampton

British Library Cataloguing in Publication Data
Powell, Trevor
  Head Injury: Practical Guide
  I.Title
  617.51044

ISBN 0-86388-126-2

CONTENTS

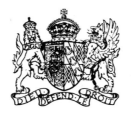

FOREWORD
BY HRH THE PRINCESS OF WALES

A head injury in the family will affect all members of that family. Any head injury resulting in damage to the brain may cause long-term or even permanent changes in a person's ability to speak, to think, to move around, to perform everyday activities independently. Perhaps most difficult to accept can be changes in the personality and behaviour of a long-known and loved family member. The prospect of coping with these changes must be a daunting one for any mother, wife, son, or any other relative, and indeed for many professional care-givers.

Trevor Powell's account of head injury makes this complex disability clear and understandable. However, this is much more than a text book. Families and professionals will find much to help them practically in their task of helping the head-injured person to help themselves. People with head injury too will find encouragement and guidance.

As Patron of Headway National Head Injuries Association, I have had the opportunity to see the work being done, both nationally and in the local Headway Groups. I am sure that this book will be invaluable to people with head injuries and those concerned with their rehabilitation.

Diana

HEADWAY

Headway National Head Injuries Association was founded in March 1980. Its aims are:

- ▶ to increase public awareness and understanding of head injury;
- ▶ to participate in activities that will reduce the incidence of head injury;
- ▶ to provide information and support for people with head injuries, their relatives and carers;
- ▶ to promote co-ordinated multidisciplinary approaches to head-injury screening, acute care, assessment, rehabilitation and community re-entry, with clear accountability at all stages;
- ▶ to assist people with head injuries to return to community living, including access to appropriate accommodation, social outlets and productive activity.

To further these ends, Headway operates a telephone and mail information service answering hundreds of enquiries each week. It publishes a range of booklets on relevant topics, most of which are aimed specifically at a non-professional readership. Study days and conferences are also organized and an annual 'National Head Injuries Week' is co-ordinated in order to raise public awareness of the impact of traumatic brain injury. Headway is involved with several initiatives to prevent head injury.

Headway's self-help groups are a source of strength and support to people with head injuries and their families. There are now 106 local groups affiliated to Headway, 33 of which manage Headway Houses. These are specialized day centres where people with head injury can go, to find understanding, occupation, enjoyment and to regain self-esteem.

The addresses of the national Headway organizations can be found at the back of the book.

TREVOR POWELL

Trevor Powell BA (Hons), MSC, AFBPs, CPsychol is an experienced practising consultant clinical psychologist, who works for the health service in the field of neuropsychological rehabilitation and adult mental health. He has been involved with the Headway charity for the last 10 years, being chairman of Headway Berkshire and a director of Headway National Head Injuries Association.

He has published research and written articles on head injury and on various forms of therapy. He is the co-author of *Anxiety and Stress Management* (Routledge, 1990) and the author of *The Mental Health Handbook* (Winslow Press Ltd, 1992). Trevor is married and lives in Berkshire.

PREFACE

The hidden psychological, social and emotional problems created by head injury have, until recently, been largely ignored, misjudged or dismissed. These long-term problems are not of a medical nature, but are concerned with the adjustment of individuals and families to the realities of life after head injury. This book attempts to provide a practical down-to-earth guide through some of these difficult areas. The book is written for families, carers, people who have experienced head injury and a variety of workers in the field. Those professionals include doctors, nurses, occupational therapists, speech therapists, physiotherapists, psychologists, social workers, solicitors, teachers, care assistants, volunteers and anybody else who has contact with people suffering from a head injury.

The book aims to work on three levels. Firstly, it is a collection of people's personal experiences, stories, anecdotes and comments. It is hoped that the reader will find some comfort and reassurance in knowing that others have experienced similar problems. Secondly, the book is a compilation of factual information and research, delivered in a non-technical, jargon-free way, to give the reader greater understanding of head injury. Thirdly, the book offers specific guidance and practical advice on ways of dealing with difficulties connected with head injury. Of course, there are no absolute answers, and certainly no solutions, but I hope this book goes some way to providing helpful pointers and insights into what is an immensely difficult situation, particularly for the sufferers and their families.

My involvement with head injury has largely been inspired by Roseanne Barnett, mother of a head-injured son and the co-ordinator of our local Headway support group and Headway Day Centre. Her voice has been echoing in my head while I have written this book. I hope I have managed to convey some of her wisdom. I do not profess to have first-hand experience of either the struggle of the person with the head injury, or the emotional turmoil of the family, but I feel I have gained an understanding of head injury by listening to many stories of great courage and determination during my 10 years' involvement with our district clinical psychology service and Headway. It is this information that I would like to share.

As the majority of people who experience head injury are males, and to avoid the rather cumbersome non-sexist language 'she/he', I have used the pronouns 'he' and 'him' throughout the book.

Trevor Powell

ACKNOWLEDGEMENTS

Special thanks to all those people who have shared their stories and experiences, on which this book is based. Thanks to all those involved in Headway, who have read various drafts of the book and made comments – Jenny Sheridan, Barbara Weston, Katie Fields, Roseanne Barnett, Margaret Bray and Sarah Durrant. I would also like to express my appreciation to the various authors who produced the numerous Headway booklets which have been a cornerstone of this work. Thanks also to West Berkshire Health Authority and in particular Alistair Keddie, District Clinical Psychologist, for allowing me time to work on this project. A special word of thanks to Andrea Rakowicz, who mastered the mysteries of the word processor and typed the manuscript so diligently; her daily encouragement and enthusiasm sustained me through difficult times. Finally particular thanks to my wife, Meriel, who corrected my English and provided me with the encouragement and love to keep me going.

INFORMATION ABOUT HEAD INJURY: SETTING THE SCENE

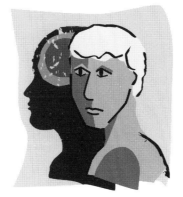

Chapter 1

INTRODUCTION

A head injury can happen to anyone. It does not matter who you are or what you do. This injury can range from a bump on the head, which leaves minimal long-term consequences, to a catastrophic injury which irrevocably alters the whole pattern of a person's life. These injuries happen in a matter of seconds. Anyone who has had a head injury has a different story to tell, in terms of both the injury and of the residual problems and outcome. No two stories are alike. What most have in common is that individuals and families confront intolerable difficulties, which necessitate plumbing the depths of their own resources and emotions. The personal qualities of love, fortitude, patience, faith and courage are severely tested, often highlighting the indomitable nature of the human spirit.

This book is meant to be a guide, offering some help for those whose life has been affected by head injury, and for those who work with people who have suffered head injury. There are no magical cures or short cuts; rather there is a long, difficult journey towards coping. Understanding more about that journey, and the potential pitfalls, and sharing the experiences of others who have trodden that road before, can surely only help. Before embarking on our journey, let us set the scene by telling seven very brief stories, to give a picture of the variety of different types of injury, and the varied after-effects and degrees of recovery.

SEVEN STORIES

Paul, a 30-year-old painter and decorator, fell from scaffolding and sustained a severe injury. Two years later he still has not returned to work and spends most of his time at home. He plays on his home computer but often has to ask his nine-year-old daughter for help in getting into the programme. He looks perfectly well, but has severe memory problems, finds it very difficult to learn anything new, and is very moody and quick to anger. He refers to himself as one of the 'walking wounded'.

Neil used to love messing about with motorbikes. His injury occurred when he was knocked off his bike by a lorry. He has now lost his job because of problems with memory, organizing and planning. He also has a lowered tolerance of frustration. Last week, for the first time, he tried to work on his bike, taking it apart and cleaning it, but he became so frustrated when he was unable to reassemble it that he flew into a rage and smashed up his beloved machine with a hammer.

Peggy fell backwards onto concrete when a large dog jumped up at her. The doctors at the local hospital told her to go home and rest in bed for a day. Three months later she still had enormous difficulty coping with her job as an executive because of excessive tiredness and poor concentration. It was only after 12 months that she felt that she was 'back to her old self'.

George was involved in a fight outside a night club, where he was hit on the head with a hammer. He now works as a gardener and plays darts for his local pub team, but he finds it impossible to add up the scores in the way he used to.

Sarah was planning to go to art school. She accepted a lift from a friend who had been drinking after a party and found herself in hospital for six months. She can still paint from her wheelchair but her tremor means that she cannot draw a straight line. Although she still enjoys going to galleries she invariably forgets where she has been and what she has seen.

William was just 18 when he was involved in a serious road traffic accident. He spent two weeks in intensive care. His mother, sitting at his bedside, was told, "It's touch and go and, if he survives, don't expect too much. He might be a vegetable." Three years later William has just successfully completed the first year of a university degree course in archaeology and, amazingly, appears to have few residual symptoms.

Jonathan banged his head in a school rugby match. For the last 10 years he has worked, but has never managed to hold down a job for more than six months. His expectations are unrealistic and he does not recognize and accept a number of his problems. Because of his frustration, he has developed a serious drinking problem. He is now living and working in a Christian community.

LETTER FROM A PARENT

Let us consider a letter written by a father whose 19-year-old son had a head injury, in order to highlight, firstly, how a head injury can affect the whole family, and secondly how it can be greatly misunderstood, even by professionals. This 'open letter' was written as a plea to all those concerned, and captures a number of common themes which will arise throughout this book. The letter was entitled, 'The Lucky Ones'.

"To whom it may concern

'Our plea to the medical world is that although you see us as the lucky ones we still need help and understanding. You see, it does not feel lucky to have a head injury or to have a relative who has one. We appreciate that many people die or have serious brain damage as a result of road accidents, but our experience is of one of "the lucky ones" who needs understanding and guidance — things which we have found to be generally lacking.

'To family and friends we would say that, although outwardly "the lucky one" appears well, inside so much is wrong. Understanding, love, time, patience and gentle encouragement are all needed in large measures.

' "The lucky one" does not feel lucky, nor does the family hit by shock struggling to look after him. Confusion, sadness and desperation are all felt by "the lucky one" who feels different from the way he felt before the accident, but does not know why. The family is also confused, frightened and unsure how to help.

'Life for the injured is harder than usual — a real struggle in fact as he tries to sort out his thoughts, agonisingly slowly, and remembering even little day-to-day things is sometimes impossible; but he looks so normal that no one understands or seems to care. He is expected to act and think the way he did before the accident, but he just can't. On top of that he feels so utterly exhausted. Everything is such hard work. Due to the confusion and inability to cope, friends shy away until he is left on his own. He longs for their understanding but he looks so normal and when he says he is having trouble with his memory, people reply, "So do I, I am always forgetting things", or if he says he is exhausted he receives the reply, "Oh yes, I feel tired all the time too." But it's different for the head-injured, who eventually says nothing about his memory or exhaustion, and retreats into himself. Of course his injury does not show like a broken leg in plaster — people make allowances for anyone in that condition. He is not seeking sympathy or pity, only understanding or at least some attempt to understand, so that people might realise why he acts the way he does. He can't put into words the way he feels, but he knows he does not feel right. He is afraid of being left alone in case he can't cope, he panics in crowds, and is afraid to travel on the road — after all it was a road accident that made him feel the way he does; but to the world he is a "lucky one".

'He finds new tasks difficult to accomplish. He remembers things learnt before the accident, but learning new things and remembering things he is told is virtually impossible. Likewise, making decisions, even simple ones, is an insurmountable task. He can't explain why these things appear so difficult for him, but people do not understand because he looks so normal.

'To the member of the nursing staff who gets cross with a head-injured patient when he does something he has been told not to do, or forgets to do something he was told to do, we say, "Please don't get cross, the patient really can't help it and he needs your understanding."

'To the doctors who say he will be back to normal in a few weeks and should be able to return to work then, we say, "Please find out more about how head injuries affect patients, and the time it can take to recover, even partially, from those injuries." Families of the injured hang on to every word spoken by a doctor — after all he or she is expected to have some knowledge of how the injuries might affect the patient, so it is very important that doctors choose their words carefully, do not build up false hopes for the family, and do not make statements that with hindsight even the layman can see are very misleading.

'We would also ask the medical world, "Where is the post-hospitalisation care?" as, in our experience, the patient is sent out from hospital and expected to cope on his own. His only link with anyone "medical" is his GP who, with the best will in the world, is unable to offer any help other than to see the patient and ask rudimentary questions without providing any answers or details of where assistance might be sought. Bearing in mind the number of head injuries which occur annually, we were surprised that there appeared to be no one to turn to for help; at least, if there was, then neither the hospital nor the GP was aware of such a person or organization.

'Our son returned to work, but even now only part-time, and when his job was changed he felt he could not cope. That situation has still not been resolved yet.

'It has been two years now and our son is still not one hundred per cent well; the last two years have been a nightmare for the whole family and we are not through it yet. If only we had known more about what to expect and how to cope when our son was discharged from hospital. It has been a shock and a frightening experience for us all. Our daughter was diagnosed as suffering from post-traumatic stress and was put in touch with a social worker who involved the whole family and, through his sympathetic attitude, was able to help us all.

'Six months ago we at last found a professional interested in head injury, although he worked in the neighbouring health district. It was a relief and a tremendous help to find someone who knew how we all felt. The Headway publications he offered us were also greatly reassuring. Our sincere thanks go out to all those who have listened, tried to understand, and did not tell us we were the lucky ones. Time does heal.'

A SILENT EPIDEMIC

Over the last two decades the number of people suffering from head injuries has increased so dramatically that it has been described as a 'silent epidemic'. The first reason for this is the enormous medical advances, high-quality technology and improved emergency services, which mean that more people are surviving. It is estimated that, as late as the 1970s, 90 per cent of all severe head-injured patients died; now the majority survive. The single most important factor in reducing deaths after head injury is the newly acquired technical ability of doctors to recognize and treat blood clots in the brain. The second reason would seem to be that we live in an age of speed and risk. Think of how many more motorways exist and the increased number of cars there are on the roads. It could be said that the speed of life has increased, people travel more, and as quickly as possible. The result of these two factors is that more people are having head injuries, more people are being kept alive and more people are walking around with the residual after-effects of head injury. The magnitude of the problem is seen to be even greater when we realize that a large percentage of survivors are adolescents and young adults with relatively normal life expectancies. It is also undoubtedly true that, although there has been a dramatic increase in head injuries, there has not been the corresponding increase in post-hospital health care. Therefore this means that the majority of people with head injury do not receive the care they need after the acute medical emergency is over.

FACTS ABOUT HEAD INJURY

I   It is estimated that one million people in Britain attend hospital every year as a result of having a head injury.

2   Every year, out of every 100,000 of the population, there is likely to be between 10 and 15 people suffering a severe head injury, 15–20 people suffering a moderate head injury and between 250 and 300 people with a mild head injury.

3   One family in every 300 will be affected by the long-term effects of head injury. That is a prevalence rate of 100–150 disabled survivors per 100,000 of the population at any one time, or more than 120,000 people in the UK suffering from the long-term effects of severe head injury. This figure is increasing every year, as the victims of head injury tend to be young, with a normal life expectancy.

4 In the USA there have been more fatalities from head injury over the last 12 years than in all the wars in which the USA has ever fought.

5 Males are two to three times more likely to have a head injury than females. In the age range 15–29, males are five times more likely to do so.

6 The age groups most at risk for head injury are 15–29 and over 65 years.

7 Road traffic accidents account for 40–50 per cent of all injuries, and are most commonly associated with severe injuries. Domestic and industrial accidents and falls account for 20–30 per cent, sports and recreational injuries for 10–15 per cent, and assaults for 10 per cent.

8 Some 90 per cent of all those who have a severe head injury make a good physical recovery. This means that their disability is effectively hidden.

9 Cycling injuries account for approximately 20 per cent of all head injuries in children. Riders with helmets have an 85 per cent reduction in risk of head injury.

10 Relatives of people who have had a head injury report that the 10 most difficult problems are: personality changes, slowness, poor memory, irritability, bad temper, tiredness, depression, rapid mood changes, tension and anxiety, and threats of violence.

11 Individuals with a personality inclined towards 'risk', or 'trying something new', obviously tend to be at greater risk. Other high-risk groups include those who have previously had a head injury and those who abuse alcohol.

12 The majority of head injuries are preventable.

WHAT DOES THE BRAIN DO?

To understand anything about the effects of a head injury we need to have some understanding of what the brain does and how it works. What does the brain do? The answer to that question is *everything*! Our brains do all our thinking, reasoning and planning, store all our memories, control all our physical actions, such as walking, talking, hearing, seeing, eating, sleeping and breathing, and control all our feelings. Our brains are our control and command centre connected by the spinal cord and a network of nerves to our whole body, from the tips of our toes to the top of our head. They are far more complicated than the most sophisticated computer system in the world. Under normal circumstances we do not give this 'silent service' a second thought. We simply live our lives and take for granted that our brains function smoothly. It is only when tragedy strikes that we become more aware.

Let us take an everyday example to illustrate how our brains work. Imagine you are walking along the street and you meet a friend whom you have not seen for a couple of years. You would:

- expect to see him,
- expect to walk smoothly towards him,
- expect to recognize his face,
- expect to remember his name,
- match the face to the name,
- remember a vast amount of personal information and adjust your welcome accordingly,
- speak to him,
- listen and understand what he says,
- experience a pleasurable emotion, or the reverse, at the meeting,
- remember the meeting for at least a day or two,
- remember it for the rest of your life, if the meeting was significant.

For each of these hardly considered thoughts, actions and emotions, different areas of our brain must be involved, activating millions of nerve cells. The effects of a head injury may mean that a number of these processes, which we take for granted, do not occur.

A BASIC ANATOMY LESSON

Over the last hundred years, a huge library of knowledge about the way the brain works has evolved. There follows an attempt to summarize this knowledge as concisely as possible.

The brain weighs around three pounds (1.3 kg) and is completely surrounded by a hard, protective, rounded shell of bone, known as the *skull* or *cranium*. The important thing to remember about the skull is that, for some strange reason, underneath the front of the skull there are a number of bony ridges. When the soft tissue of the brain is shaken around these ridges have the unfortunate effect of lacerating and damaging the underside of the front of the brain. On the floor of the skull is a hole where the lower part of the brain or *brain stem* is connected to the *spinal cord*, and from there to the whole of the nervous system and the rest of the body (see Figure 1). The brain stem is rather like a thick telecommunications cable, with countless nerve fibres like wires, carrying messages backwards and forwards. This brain stem area is also known to control such bodily functions as wakefulness, consciousness, tiredness, heartbeat and blood pressure. Damage to this area is thought to cause concussion and loss of consciousness.

The texture of the brain is rather like soft blancmange, but it is held together in the skull by a number of layers of membrane called the *dura*, *pia* and *arachnoid*. Between the pia and arachnoid membranes is the subarachnoid space, in which run the *blood vessels* supplying and draining the brain. Like any organ, the brain is dependent on blood from the heart, and is criss-crossed by a network of large arteries, which divide into progressively smaller branches. When the brain is shaken about in a head injury, these vessels tear and bleed. As we get older our blood vessels become more brittle and more likely to tear if shaken around. This bleeding leads to a build-up of blood clots, which pressurizes and damages the delicate tissue of the brain. The brain in its membranous sack floats in a sea of *cerebrospinal fluid*, which fills in all the gaps around the brain and offers some protection and cushioning. Just behind the brain

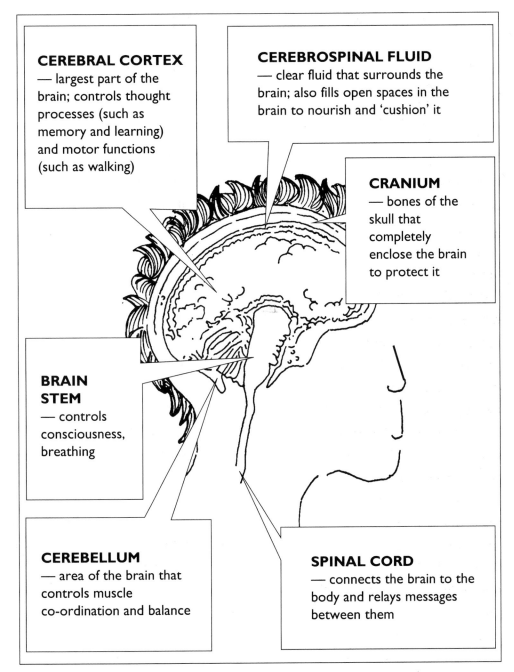

CEREBRAL CORTEX
— largest part of the brain; controls thought processes (such as memory and learning) and motor functions (such as walking)

CEREBROSPINAL FLUID
— clear fluid that surrounds the brain; also fills open spaces in the brain to nourish and 'cushion' it

CRANIUM
— bones of the skull that completely enclose the brain to protect it

BRAIN STEM
— controls consciousness, breathing

CEREBELLUM
— area of the brain that controls muscle co-ordination and balance

SPINAL CORD
— connects the brain to the body and relays messages between them

Figure 1 *Anatomy of the brain*

stem sits a curved lump of tissue called the *cerebellum*; this area regulates all our fine motor co-ordination involved in such skills as balancing, moving quickly and gracefully, dancing, threading a needle, or climbing a ladder.

The largest part of the brain is known as the *cerebral cortex* and is shaped like a large wrinkled walnut (see Figure 2). Resembling a walnut, it is divided into two halves and joined by a bridge in the middle. The two halves are known as the right and left cerebral hemispheres. It is known that the right side controls the left side of our body and the left side controls the right side of our body. Damage only to the right side may affect movement in the left arm and leg or hearing in the left ear. There is also evidence that for most people the left hemisphere contains the language centres involving speech, while the right hemisphere tends to control non-language, spatial skills such as drawing or musical ability. If a person received injuries only to the left side of the brain, by for example having a stroke, it is likely that his speech would be affected, as would the ability to move the right-hand side of the body. Strokes tend to affect a specific area, whereas a head injury due to a road traffic accident usually involves more general damage.

The make-up of the brain consists of billions of microscopic nerve cells. Under a powerful microscope these cells look like small dots with a network of hair-like tentacles (axons or dendrites; see Figure 3). They communicate with each other by passing electrical and chemical impulses between these tentacles. Highly complex patterns of communication, or pathways, build up as the brain develops throughout childhood. The effect of a head injury on this delicate substance is similar to that of vigorously shaking a plate of blancmange — it shears and tears, disrupting those pathways of communication.

Apart from dividing into a left and right hemisphere, the cerebral cortex can be further divided into a number of areas known as lobes (see Figure 2). The *frontal lobe* is the area behind the forehead and is heavily involved in intellectual activities such as planning and organizing, as well as being involved in personality and the control of emotions and behaviour. Just behind and below the frontal lobes are the *temporal lobes,*

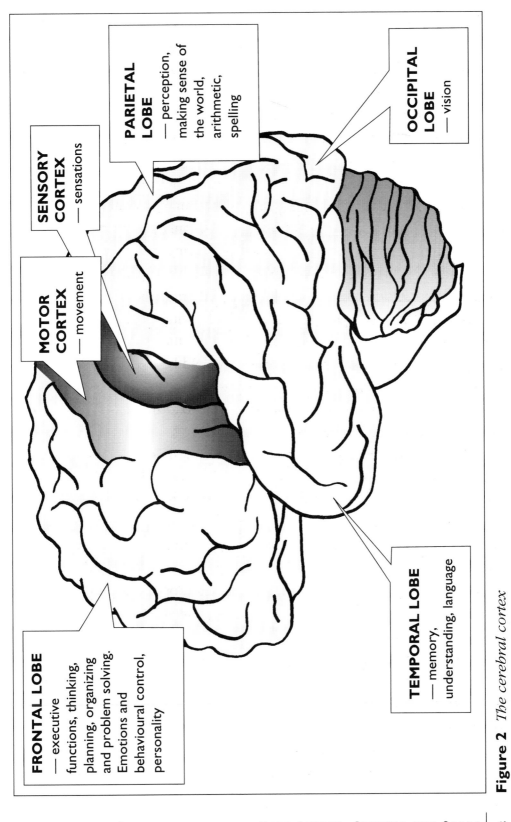

Figure 2 *The cerebral cortex*

SENSORY CORTEX
— sensations

PARIETAL LOBE
— perception, making sense of the world, arithmetic, spelling

OCCIPITAL LOBE
— vision

MOTOR CORTEX
— movement

TEMPORAL LOBE
— memory, understanding, language

FRONTAL LOBE
— executive functions, thinking, planning, organizing and problem solving. Emotions and behavioural control, personality

nestled behind the ears; this area holds the bulk of our memories and our ability to understand things and speak. At the back of the brain above the ears sit the *parietal lobes*, which have an important role to play in our ability to understand spatial relationships and to read and write. Between the frontal and parietal lobes are areas which control movement and

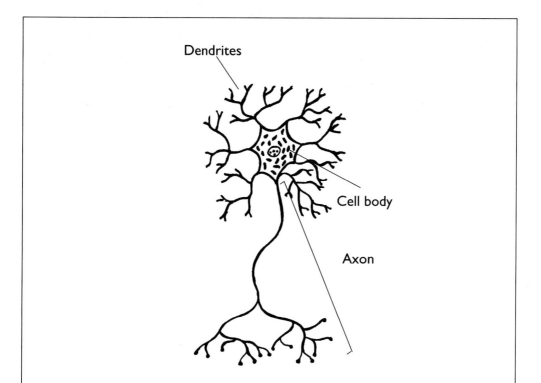

1   All nerve cells, or neurones, are the same. They have a cell body which sprouts dendrites, which receive impulses, and axons which transmit impulses.
2   Cells pass information along their fibres in the form of electrical and chemical messages.
3   Each individual cell or neurone is in contact with 1–2,000 other nerve cells.
4   The brain is made up of about 1,000,000,000,000 nerve cells.

Figure 3 *The nerve cell*

sensation. At the very back of the head are the *occipital lobes,* which are responsible for sight: injury to this area can cause partial or complete blindness.

Hidden in the middle of this walnut-like cerebral cortex are a number of small white nerve centres, collectively known as the *diencephalon.* In this area lies the small pea-sized *hypothalamus,* which controls appetite regulation, sexual arousal, thirst and temperature control, and some aspects of memory. Close to this area is another important set of nuclei, referred to as the *limbic system.* Damage to this area can play havoc with emotions, leaving the individual with dramatic and sudden mood swings.

WHAT HAPPENS IN A HEAD INJURY

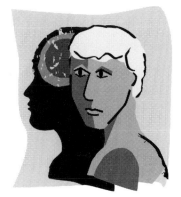

Chapter 2

THE INJURY ITSELF

The highly sophisticated computer, our brain, which controls our whole being and every action, is not resting immobile on a desk in somebody's office, but is constantly moving around. It hurtles down motorways at 70 miles an hour, and to a certain extent is shaken, banged and knocked about without harm. However damage can be caused if we are too rough with it. A head injury can be defined as 'damage to living brain tissue that is initially caused by external mechanical forces'. This contrasts with brain injury caused by internal events such as blood vessels bursting (strokes), growth of tumours, viruses or development of diseases.

The most common causes of head injury are road traffic accidents, domestic or industrial accidents, sports and recreational injuries, and assaults. A head injury is usually characterized by periods of altered consciousness (coma) and/or periods of amnesia; these may be very brief, lasting minutes or hours, or much longer, spanning weeks or even months. The effect of the injury is tissue damage which can impair physical, mental and emotional abilities.

A head injury is usually not just one injury but a series of injuries. The first injury occurs at the time of the impact and is the direct damage to the brain. The second injury occurs in the minutes afterwards and is due to lack of oxygen to the brain. The third injury occurs in the next days, up to a month, and is the result of bleeding, bruising and swelling which damages brain tissue.

The First Injury

The first injury is the tissue damage due to the direct impact. There are two types of direct impact injuries, which are either penetrating or closed head injuries (see Figure 4).

A *penetrating injury*, which is comparatively rare, occurs when an object, such as a bullet or an ice pick, fractures the skull, enters the brain and rips into the soft tissue in its path. These injuries usually damage relatively localized areas of the brain, which results in quite specific

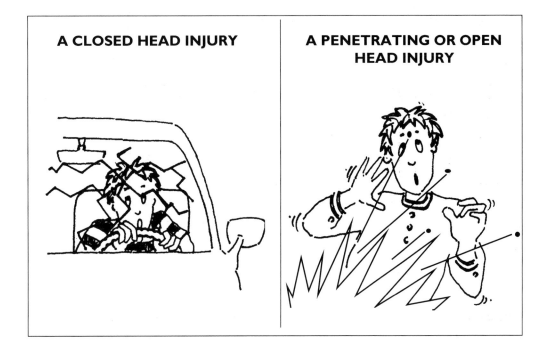

| A CLOSED HEAD INJURY | A PENETRATING OR OPEN HEAD INJURY |

Figure 4 *Different types of head injury*

disabilities.

A *closed head injury*, which is much more common, occurs when the brain is either accelerated, decelerated or rotated very quickly, usually after colliding with another object, for example the windscreen of a car. Damage occurs because of the violent movement, not because of the presence of a foreign object within the brain. As described in Chapter 1, the brain resembles soft blancmange, in a bag, encased in the hard bony skull, with rough edges. If you violently shake a blancmange on a plate, shear lines or cracks appear, or the top part may lag behind the base, or even fly off. When the brain is violently shaken around, this movement damages the delicate connection between the nerve cell tentacles (axons and dendrites), breaking up communication pathways. This is called diffuse axonal damage. Violent movement also causes the soft brain to be lacerated along the sharp bony ridges on the underside of the front of the skull, often damaging the most important parts of the brain, the temporal and frontal lobes. With the acceleration or deceleration injuries sustained in car accidents, the brain smashes forwards and then backwards, rebounding against the wall of the skull, causing damage and bruising to both the front and back of the brain. A further effect of violent shaking within the brain is referred to as 'the cheese-cutter effect'; this happens when the large blood vessels, which are relatively well tethered, sever adjacent tissue, as the more mobile soft brain structure moves by.

The Second Injury

The second injury is concerned with an interruption in the oxygen supply to the brain, carried in the blood, during the immediate minutes after the accident. Although the brain is only 2 per cent of the whole body's weight it consumes 20 per cent of the oxygen carried by the blood. If this blood supply is interrupted even for two or three minutes, the brain cells are starved and will die. This can happen if there is extensive bleeding which reduces blood pressure, if there are chest injuries or if the windpipe is blocked by vomited food or blood. This absolute need of oxygen to the brain is the reason why an ambulanceman will make sure the breathing is free and easy immediately on arrival at the scene of an accident and will set up an emergency blood transfusion if necessary. Later on the patient may be put on a ventilator, in the intensive care unit, to safeguard the breathing and oxygen supply to the brain. Interrupted oxygen supply to the brain is called hypoxia (or anoxia).

The Third Injury

The third type of injury occurs in the hours and days after the original accident. These injuries consist of bleeding, bruising and swelling of the brain, and the development of blood clots.

The brain bruises and swells like any other part of the body. This is due to the tearing and bleeding of very small blood vessels and the leakage of other body fluids into this area. This swelling is a problem because the brain is enclosed in the hard, unyielding skull. As the brain swells, pressure builds up and the soft tissue of the brain is squeezed against the walls of the skull, causing damage. The swollen brain also squeezes the main arteries, causing blood circulation to be impaired or stopped. If the blood circulation stops the patient dies. This pressure inside the skull is known as 'intracranial pressure', or ICP, and has to be very carefully monitored. To keep the intracranial pressure down, brain swelling must be kept to a minimum. One way of doing this involves making sure that the brain has plenty of oxygen, and that blood pressure is kept high. This can be achieved by putting the patient on a ventilator which controls breathing. A second measure is to control strictly the amount of water and salt in the body to reduce the flow of tissue fluid into the brain.

Blood clots occur when the larger blood vessels and arteries are torn, and enough blood escapes to form a pool of blood which compresses and damages the brain around it. It also increases intracranial pressure, and if the bleeding does not stop it can push this pressure over the limit and cause death. These clots, or 'haematomas', can sometimes occur after quite minor injuries, and this is why patients are often kept in hospital for observation, until the risk of a clot is over. They can occur either in the brain itself (an intracerebral clot) or in the space between the brain and the skull (a subdural or extradural clot, depending on which side of the thick dura membrane it occurs).

Two further unusual conditions that can occur a week or more later are known as 'chronic subdural haematomas', and 'post-traumatic hydrocephalus'. The chronic subdural haematoma is a slow-growing blood clot that is too small to be detected at first, but grows over weeks until it pressurizes the brain. Post-traumatic hydrocephalus occurs when circulation around the brain is blocked by the scarring which follows brain injury. The fluid accumulates within the brain and the intracranial pressure rises. Both of these complications can be treated quite simply by a small operation, which involves cutting a small trap-door in the skull to relieve the pressure until the swelling dies down.

Damage to the Skull

In most closed head injuries there is not any specific damage to the skull. If there is, the bone of the skull mends itself quite quickly. The reason for patients being admitted to hospital with this kind of injury is really a precaution to anticipate further injuries, such as infections. A fractured skull which is usually a crack in the round dome of the head is described as a 'compound fracture'. If the skull is broken so much that there are fragments projecting inwards, perhaps into the brain, this is called a 'depressed fracture'. In both of these cases there is an increased risk of infection and possible epilepsy.

If the fracture involves the bone of the forehead or the roof of the nose, the fluid around the brain (cerebrospinal fluid) may escape and run down the nose. One important consequence is that bacteria may get in and cause meningitis, but this can be remedied by antibiotics. Fracture of the skull base also injures the nerves which leave the brain, causing a disturbance of sight, hearing or some other function of the face. If the injury has caused a gap in the skull, after a few months, when the wound has healed and all chances of infection have gone, a bone graft or a metal plate may be put in to fill the hole. The vast majority of skull fractures heal themselves without any medical intervention being necessary.

COMA

Whether it be for a few seconds or a few weeks, the usual immediate effect of a head injury is a loss of consciousness. Coma or concussion is not fully understood but is thought to be associated with activities in the brain stem. Coma can be defined as a state of depressed consciousness where the person is unresponsive to the outside world. There are different levels of coma, ranging from a very deep one, where the patient shows no response to pain, to more shallow levels, where the patient will respond to pain by movement or opening eyes, to still shallower levels where the patient will make some response to speech.

The Glasgow Coma Scale is a very simple, easy-to-administer technique, which is universally used to rate the severity of coma via the patient's ability to open his eyes, move and speak. A patient is assigned a number in each of three categories: eye opening, motor response and verbal response. The minimum possible score is three and the maximum possible score is 15. The more severe the injury, the lower his performance, and the lower the number he is assigned. A very low number suggests a very serious injury, and little likelihood of total recovery.

Glasgow Coma Scale

Eye opening

Spontaneous 4

To speech 3

To pain 2

None 1

Best motor response

Obeys commands 6

Moves within the general locale 5

Withdraws 4

Abnormal muscle bending and flexing 3

Involuntary muscle straightening and extending 2

None 1

Verbal response

Is orientated 5

Confused conversation 4

Inappropriate words 3

Incomprehensible sounds 2

None 1

Minimum score 3   Maximum score 15

Recovery from a coma is a gradual process, starting with eyes opening, then responding to pain, and then responding to speech. People do not just wake up from a coma, and say, "Where am I?" as sometimes represented in films. The length of coma is one of the most accurate predictors of the severity of residual symptoms. The longer the coma, the greater the likelihood of residual symptoms, particularly physical disabilities. Hospital staff using the Glasgow Coma Scale can monitor improvement as the patient's score moves from very low numbers such as four, five and six to higher scores. A score of 14 indicates that the patient is out of the coma, and usually in a state where he is fully conscious but his everyday memory is not working.

Trust Your Instincts — A Mother's Story

"It's a strange thing to say, but ever since Alistair was born I've had a strong feeling that something terrible was going to happen to him — there was something in the wind. As a teenager he was a bit of a tearaway and caused us a great deal of heartache. The feeling that something was going to happen got stronger as he got older. One day I heard loud ambulance bells ringing, and I just knew that they were for Alistair, and so it proved to be. He had been in a road traffic accident and was in a coma for four weeks. The coma was a living nightmare for the whole family. The doctors gave him little chance of surviving, but deep down I knew he'd come through it. A member of our family sat at his bedside throughout the coma; we worked shifts, just talking to him as we normally would and holding his hand. In the second week, I was at home preparing a meal and I had a very strong feeling that there was something wrong. I rang the hospital expressing my concern. The nurses tried reassuring me, but I knew they were just thinking, 'That crazy woman again.' I jumped in my car and raced to the hospital. I was right, there was something wrong. Alistair was lying there, struggling for breath, as his tracheotomy tube had become blocked. Four years on Alistair has made a good recovery, walking, talking and laughing. He still has lots of problems, but in some ways he is a much pleasanter person. The moral of my story to all women out there is, 'Trust your own instincts.'" ■

Guidelines for Managing Patients in a Coma

1   Do not talk over the head of the patient in a coma as, even though he may show no signs of responding, he may be able to understand what you are saying. Talk to the patient as you would to anybody else.

2   Exercise the patient's muscles and accessible joints, through their full range, to avoid wasting and contractures. This should be done for five to ten minutes between six and ten times a day. Ask the physiotherapist how best to do this.

3   Make the patient's room as homely and personalized as possible with photographs, a clock, a calendar and a mirror. If possible allow the patient to sit up in bed.

4   Coma stimulation programmes. There is still some controversy over the effectiveness of attempting deliberately to stimulate the person in coma. Most would say that such programmes have some beneficial effect, and they give the relatives something useful to do. It is important to consult the doctors and nurses on the ward first. Simple basic principles include the following:

  (a)   Provide stimulation to all five senses: hearing, vision, touch, taste and smell.

  (b)   Stimulation should be intense and for short periods: an ice pack on the stomach for two minutes; lemon or curry paste on a cotton bud placed on the tongue for one minute; strong perfume or garlic on a cotton bud under the nose for one minute; a familiar piece of music, or voice, for five minutes. Shine a torchlight into the patient's eyes, switched on for one to two seconds and off for five seconds, alternating for a period of three or four minutes.

  (c)   Stimulation should always be contrasted with periods of non-stimulation or rest. Implement the programme for five to ten minutes every hour, leaving the rest of the hour free of stimulation. Avoid constant noise, such as a radio blaring in the background or groups of people talking, as the patient will just 'turn off' and filter it all out.

POST-TRAUMATIC AMNESIA

Post-traumatic amnesia (PTA) is a state where the patient is conscious, lucid, on the surface appearing in touch with his surroundings and quite normal, but in fact there is something wrong as his ability to remember everyday things is not working properly. This period often follows a period of coma, although patients can experience PTA without actually being in a coma or unconscious. The patient may be able to talk to relatives, friends and nurses, but will not be able to remember these conversations or their visit a short time later. It is not uncommon for people to climb out of the wreck of a car crash and talk to their rescuers and well-wishers, but later have no memory of doing so. The patient is likely to be disoriented in time and place, not knowing the time, day, date or even year and not knowing where he is or why he is there. This period closely resembles the feeling of being awake in a dream. PTA will gradually lift, like the clouds lifting after a storm.

During this early period in hospital the patient's behaviour may well be restless, disinhibited and agitated. Uncharacteristic behaviour like swearing, shouting and masturbating in public are not unusual, but are best ignored, as seeing other people distressed may only increase his own agitation or distress. An individual cannot be held fully responsible for what he says or does in this period. This is a difficult time for relatives and nursing staff, but it is important to remember that the patient will come out of it.

Length of PTA, as with length of coma, is important, in the sense that it is the best indicator of severity of head injury. PTA is assessed by asking the patient a number of questions at regular, usually daily, intervals. The first group of questions is concerned with awareness of time, place and person: for example, "What is your name?", "Where are you now?", "What time of the day is it?", "What day of the week is it?", "What month is it?", "What year is it?" A second group of questions relates to the patient's awareness of the accident: "What was your *last* memory before the accident?", "What was your *first* memory after the accident?" A patient deep in PTA will not be able to answer these questions correctly. As he emerges from the mists of PTA the answers become more accurate and more sensible: the patient is beginning to realize what has actually happened to him.

DEGREES OF SEVERITY OF INJURY

Severity of injury ranges enormously, from banging your head on the kitchen cabinet, which leaves you feeling dizzy and sick, to a major injury which produces a coma of some months. There are a number of categories useful in distinguishing severity of injury. Each category is defined by length of time in coma, and/or period of post-traumatic amnesia. These two measures have been shown to be the best measure of eventual outcome.

Mild Head Injury

Some 75 per cent of all head injuries are considered mild, often being the result of a fall or a minor collision. Categorizing a head injury as mild means a person experiences a brief loss of consciousness (that is, less than 15 minutes), or has not been unconscious at all, with a period of post-traumatic amnesia of less than one hour. Recent research has stressed that mild injuries very often occur without a loss of consciousness. Standard neurological examinations are often normal, but newly developed, highly sophisticated brain scanners have shown that there may be some small (microscopic) nerve damage. This damage is often to frontal and temporal lobes of the brain as they smash into the bony ridges at the front underside of the skull. The incidence of these mild injuries is estimated to be between 250 and 300 per 100,000 of the population in the UK every year.

The results of mild head injury are an array of symptoms often referred to as post-concussion syndrome. Initial symptoms include nausea, headaches and dizziness, followed by impaired concentration, memory problems, difficulty processing new information, extreme tiredness, irritability, intolerance of noise and light, and lowered tolerance of alcohol. These symptoms are often followed by anxiety and depression.

Doreen — A Lady with a Mild Head Injury

Doreen acknowledged that she was a 'hard-driving lady', who in her mid-forties was trying to complete her PhD, while working full-time as a primary school teacher and being mother to two teenage children. As she cycled across the university campus absorbed in her work she failed to notice a car coming from her left. She was knocked over the handlebars of her bicycle and hit her head on the bonnet of the car. She did not lose consciousness but went along to the local hospital for a check-up, as she felt very shaken. The doctor examined her and told her that she was all right. She took his advice, went home, spent a day in bed and then tried to carry on as normal. Unfortunately she found that she could not concentrate or remember things as she could before the accident. She also felt extraordinarily tired. But she kept pushing herself, thinking that she would be all right the next day. She became increasingly upset and emotional and blamed herself for her inability to cope.

After three months her GP referred her for counselling to a clinical neuropsychologist, who showed her a Headway publication on mild head injury. She felt greatly relieved because she now understood better the cause of her problem and showed the pamphlet to all the teachers in the staff room to help them better to understand. For the rest of the school year, she reluctantly opted out of the extra-curricular activities, consciously tried to reduce her stress levels, and most evenings would go to bed early, as she usually felt exhausted. In time she felt progressively better and gradually took on an increased workload at school. She now feels 'back to her old self'. ■

A commonly occurring problem is that the patient may return home, or even begin work after a few days, and find that he just cannot cope. Because the mental impairments are rather subtle, and often nobody has warned him of the possibility of difficulties, the patient may feel frustrated and blame himself for his incompetence. The patient and relatives simply do not understand what has happened to them. It is important for patients to be warned about possible adverse reactions and to plan accordingly. This might include being cautioned against immediate return to work and advised to abstain from alcohol, or contact sports (eg. Rugby, Football) which increase the risk of a second injury.

One study showed that almost one-third of persons with a mild head injury were not working full-time three months after receiving the injury, although other studies have been much more optimistic. Difficulties are certainly made worse if the person has a mentally demanding job where there is a low margin of error. The general conclusion seems to be that the vast majority of people who experience a mild head injury make a full recovery, usually after 3–4 months. However there does appear to be a very small subgroup whose recovery is not so good.

Moderate Head Injury

A moderate head injury is defined as a loss of consciousness of between 15 minutes and six hours, and a period of post-traumatic amnesia of up to 24 hours. The patient can be kept in hospital overnight for observation during the acute phase and then discharged if there are no further obvious medical injuries. Like those with a mild head injury, patients with a moderate injury are likely to suffer from a number of residual symptoms. The most commonly reported symptoms include tiredness, headaches, dizziness, difficulties with thinking, attention, memory, planning, organizing and concentration, word-finding problems and irritability. These symptoms are accompanied by understandable worry and anxiety — this can be particularly pronounced if the patient has not been warned that these problems are likely to arise. If the patient expects to be perfectly well within a few days, and symptoms are still prominent after a few weeks, they may worry, or feel guilty, which then has the effect of creating

The Unseen Injury — Mild and Moderate Head Injury

1 Up to 95 per cent of all head injuries are minor (either mild or moderate). Usually the person has no outward signs of injury, hence the term 'the unseen injury'.

2 The head is not always struck in a minor head injury. Often the injury can occur as a result of sudden violent motions, such as a whiplash injury, being shaken, or a fall.

3 Recently developed MRI scanners, which take images of the brain, can often identify damaged nerve fibres, which have been stretched, torn or bruised in a minor head injury.

4 Minor head injuries are common in sports. Boxing is the only sport where participants deliberately try to inflict a head injury on each other.

5 Most people receive no follow-up after visiting the casualty department of a hospital. The following advice might be helpful:

(a) It is likely that headaches, excessive tiredness, concentration, memory and emotional problems, and a reduced tolerance of alcohol will be experienced. For the vast majority of people these symptoms will gradually disappear over the coming weeks, or possibly months.

(b) The brain needs to recover without undue stress being placed on it. Mental activity should be restricted to routine tasks that are undemanding. The day should be planned to conserve energy, including more sleep if it is needed. Major decisions, changes of routine, or other stresses should be avoided or postponed. The art of saying 'no' should be cultivated.

(c) If possible, it is advisable to delay an immediate return to work, particularly if the job involves a high level of stress and only a small margin of error. Eventual return should be gradual.

(d) Educate others, including employers, about the subtle hidden problems of minor head injury. Do not fall victim to accusations of malingering or imaginary symptoms.

a vicious circle of worry, leading to more symptoms and so on. A large proportion of people find that when they return to work they have difficulties and feel they are not functioning at their highest level. For the majority of people these residual symptoms gradually improve, although this can sometimes take three to four months. The incidence of this type of injury is estimated at 18 per 100,000 of the population every year in the UK.

Severe Head Injury

A severe head injury is usually defined as being a condition where the patient has been in a coma for six hours or more, or a post-traumatic amnesia of 24 hours or more. These patients are likely to be hospitalized and receive post-acute rehabilitation. Depending on the length of time in coma, these patients tend to have more serious physical deficits. The incidence of this type of injury is estimated as being between 10 and 15 per 100,000 of the UK population every year. A further category of very severe head injury is defined by a period of unconsciousness of 48 hours or more, or a period of PTA of seven days or more. The longer the length of coma and PTA, the poorer will be the outcome. However there are exceptions to this rule and, just as there is a small group of people who have a mild head injury who make a poor recovery, so there is a small group of individuals who have a severe or very severe injury who do exceptionally well.

Persistent Vegetative State

A small number of people sustain a head injury so severe that they remain in a state of coma for months and years without recovering sufficient consciousness to make any form of communication, but can breathe without mechanical assistance. They may have sleeping and waking cycles, allowing themselves to be fed, but they do not speak, follow commands or show any understanding of what has been said. Their Glasgow Coma Scale score is usually below nine. When this is the case, despite all reasonable application of rehabilitation measures for at least three years, a person may be described as being in a Persistent Vegetative

State, or PVS. There are normally just less than 100 people in the UK in PVS at any one time.

WHO'S WHO IN THE REHABILITATION TEAM

Hospitals can be confusing and frightening places for people unfamiliar with them. It helps to know something about the different professionals who are likely to be involved in a rehabilitation team.

Nurses

Nurses are trained in all aspects of general health care and will help with dressing, washing, feeding and toileting. A ward will be run by a sister or charge nurse, accompanied by a staff nurse and nursing assistants.

Doctors

A consultant will co-ordinate the day-to-day medical care, carrying out examinations and prescribing medication while the patient is in hospital. The consultant is head of a medical team and will be assisted by junior medical staff such as registrars and house officers, who will spend more time on the ward than the consultant.

Physiotherapist

The physiotherapist aims to help patients recover the ability to use their muscles and joints so they can sit or stand without losing balance, co-ordinate movements, walk and use fine hand movements. The physio-therapist will set exercises and activities for improving physical ability, and help with learning techniques for lifting and transferring from a wheelchair.

Occupational Therapist

The occupational therapist (OT) is concerned with helping develop independence in carrying out everyday tasks, such as dressing, cooking and housework. They will also help the individual develop skills which underlie these activities, such as budgeting, planning, improving thinking and finding ways around problems. They may also provide special equipment and adaptations around the home.

Clinical Psychologist

The clinical psychologist will help in assessing the patient's mental skills and weaknesses, such as memory and concentration, using specially designed tests. They may also advise on management and rehabilitation and cognitive retraining programmes in hospital and in the community. They may also provide counselling and advice on dealing with the emotional problems involved in adjustment and coping.

Social Worker

Social workers are skilled in helping families receive the practical help that is needed. They can provide information about benefits, housing, accommodation and transport. The social worker is also an experienced counsellor and is there to talk to about emotions and feelings. If, while your relative is a patient in hospital, you have not had any contact with a hospital social worker, ask for an appointment to see one.

Speech and Language Therapist

Speech and language therapists aim to help patients communicate more effectively using both the spoken and the written word. They may provide structured exercises and activities aimed at improving speech and language skills or work with other staff and relatives to improve all-round communication. The speech therapist will also have experience of communication aids.

THE ROAD TOWARDS RECOVERY

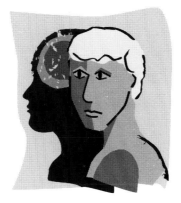

Chapter 3

THE BRAIN'S RECOVERY

Once medical stability has been achieved and the risk of secondary complications reduced, the long road towards recovery, or partial recovery, starts. We do not fully understand how the brain recovers its functioning. On the one hand, we do know that, once brain tissue is damaged, it does not spring back into life. On the other hand, we also know that the brain seems to recover quite spontaneously, especially in the first two years after injury. After that, recovery tends gradually to slow down, but nevertheless continues for years and years, as long as there is some sensory input. What is happening in the brain then?

Research suggests that, when the brain is injured, it attempts to repair itself by trying to reorganize itself. When brain injury occurs it is likely that parts of the brain that were not previously used for a particular task can be brought into operation to perform the functions previously performed by the damaged areas. In effect new pathways are being created and opened up. There is evidence to suggest that the younger the brain, the easier it is to open up these new pathways. As we get older, pathways become more established, and the brain becomes less flexible or 'plastic'. Recent theories also suggest that, when some nerve cells are damaged, but not destroyed, there can be a process of 'resprouting' amongst the tentacles (axons or dendrites) of the individual cells. This is one way that new pathways can be opened. A further theory suggests that some nerve cells are merely 'stunned', and recover their functioning after a period of suspension.

It may be useful to think of the brain in terms of the complex traffic system in a large city. Imagine the sort of disruption that would be caused by an earthquake, or a bomb going off at a particularly busy traffic intersection. For a while traffic flow would come to a complete standstill; there would be long traffic jams and general congestion. However, gradually, motorists would find new, previously unused routes around back streets and across residential areas. If the roads were not too severely damaged they might be cleared and traffic flow might continue, but at a slower pace. Traffic lights might be completely destroyed or temporarily out of action, later on being repaired. In most busy cities after a major disaster, people eventually find some way of reaching their destination. The process of recovery and rehabilitation could be viewed as the process of finding those new routes, opening up new pathways and repairing old ones.

REHABILITATION

The process of rehabilitation starts almost immediately after injury, with the provision of directed sensory stimulation, and exercising of muscles and joints. If this does not occur, contractures — stiffness — will develop. Research shows that the brain heals more effectively (grows heavier and bigger with better connections) in an 'enriched environment', ie. one which has some complexity that encourages the individual to interact. This process of formal rehabilitation, applied by professional clinicians, is likely to be limited by time constraints, but the informal rehabilitation, as applied by family members and carers, can go on for a very long time. Research suggests that the patients who make the best recovery are those whose family is actively involved, and who continue the rehabilitation process long after being discharged from formal services. Rehabilitation has two stages, the first being the formal intervention to improve the individual; the second stage is when the family and carers work to maintain that improvement. There is evidence that, once people are discharged from a formal rehabilitation environment and return to the home environment, their performance falls away unless the family have been integrated into the rehabilitation programme.

The greatest visible progress occurs in the first six months, after which improvement is often more subtle and less obvious. But progress does not stop after an arbitrary period of two years, as has been suggested in some old textbooks. Rather people continue to improve five, ten or more years after a head injury. Visible signs of progress, such as seeing a loved one, starting to walk and talk again, are very encouraging for relatives and carers, whereas later improvements, such as improving concentration or gaining more emotional control, might be less apparent. The process of rehabilitation is a long one, as is implied in the following definition by the World Health Organization at a meeting in 1986: 'Rehabilitation implies the restoration of the patient to the highest level of physical, psychological and social adaptation attainable. It includes all measures aimed at reducing the impact of the disability and handicapping conditions. It also aims at enabling disabled people to achieve optimum social integration.'

The basic requisites of good formal rehabilitation are:

(a)   to make an accurate assessment of and understand the patient's strengths and weaknesses (skills and deficits);

(b)   to plan carefully realistic goals to work towards in order to improve areas of weakness;

(c)   to break goals down into achievable steps or skills;

(d)   to teach, practise, repeat, learn and learn again those skills or small steps;

(e)   to provide directed and limited stimulation to all senses;

(f)   to offer encouragement to increase motivation;

(g)   to increase insight and aid adjustment to limitations;

(h)   to provide aids, strategies, and techniques for managing impairments where recovery is unlikely.

Unfortunately rehabilitation facilities in the UK tend to be in rather short supply, as health care resources have not kept up with this growing need. In the USA, where medical insurance companies have more of a say in dictating health care resources, over 500 rehabilitation programmes have developed over the last two decades. Good rehabilitation makes financial sense, as the more independent the patient becomes, the less reliant he is on others or the state.

Rehabilitation is often wrongly viewed as the ultimate magic cure for the after-effects of head injury. It is not. It can certainly help, but there comes a point where family and carers have to accept that the effort spent on formal rehabilitation is not bringing in equivalent returns. This is often very difficult for the family to do. It can sometimes happen that families blame the shortfall in rehabilitation services for their problems rather than accepting the limitations caused by the brain injury.

Stewart's Story — A Change of Environment Leads to Improvement

Stewart had become very overweight; he sat in his wheelchair all day. A severe aphasia meant that his speech was very limited. He had a road traffic accident 10 years ago, at the age of 28, and since then had been looked after by his elderly parents. They were kind and caring but felt guilty about Stewart's accident and tended to indulge him with sweets, cakes and treats. Stewart's father would say, "The lad gets little pleasure from life. Let him have another cake."

Sadly, Stewart's father died, leaving his mother to shoulder the burden of Stewart's care. Because he was so heavy she could not lift him from his wheelchair and so she looked out for a 'live-in carer'. Fortunately she recruited a globe-trotting Australian physiotherapist who was looking for temporary work for six months. Within five weeks of Stewart's father's death, Stewart walked very shakily into the Headway Day Centre. His steps were hesitant but this was the first time that he had ventured out of his chair since his accident ten years ago. Undoubtedly this progress was due to a change of carers, who, because they did not love him as family, did not over-indulge or over-protect him, but enabled him to stretch himself.■

THE PROCESS OF CARE

Most people who have sustained a moderate or severe head injury will be admitted to a general hospital. The patient may go to an intensive care unit, and then be moved to an open ward. This acute stage is dominated by medical input as the early goals are to save the patient's life, reduce complications and restrict the degree of brain injury. If the patient is in a coma, a sensory stimulation programme may be implemented. Physiotherapy is important to promote proper positioning and movement to prevent bed sores, weakened muscles and spasticity.

In an ideal world, once medical stability has been achieved, it is beneficial for the patient to move on to a rehabilitation unit, which may be on the campus of the general hospital or may stand alone. The goals of this unit are to help the patient reach their optimal level of independence. A multidisciplinary team should be present who can evaluate and assess the patient's needs. The physiotherapist's involvement will be to help the patient to improve physical mobility, balance, co-ordination, strength and endurance. Occupational therapists implement step-by-step programmes to help the patient improve activities of daily living such as dressing, feeding, personal hygiene, cooking and using money. The speech and language therapist is available to help the patient improve communication skills. Their role may range from advising on communicating with the head-injured person, to treating eating and swallowing disorders, to assessing aphasias. At the same time a variety of professionals, including psychologists, will be involved in cognitive rehabilitation, which means devising activities to help the patient to improve mental abilities such as memory, attention, thinking, organizing and planning. It is important at this early stage to be aware of the developments of inappropriate behaviours, which might include inappropriate touching or sexual behaviour, aggressive outbursts, excessive talking or lack of initiation. A good understanding of the principles of behaviour modification is essential. These would include the idea of reinforcement, which means understanding how adding or taking away rewards or attention can affect behaviour.

While these specific rehabilitation activities are going on, the family will need to be involved and given accurate information and counselling, to help them with adjustment of expectations and feelings concerning their loved one's disability. Similarly the person with the head injury will need counselling to help them improve self-awareness, recognize changes and adjust emotionally to their disability.

After a certain time the person with the head injury will either return home or go to another residential option (see Figure 5). Those that return home may continue with their formal rehabilitation as an out-patient. Those that are too disabled to return home may be transferred to one of a variety of residential situations, depending on their level of independence. Some people who are severely disabled and very dependent will require skilled long term nursing care. Ideally others with higher degrees of independence may move to a residential unit with some supervision, or a group home, with lower levels of supervision, and eventually to

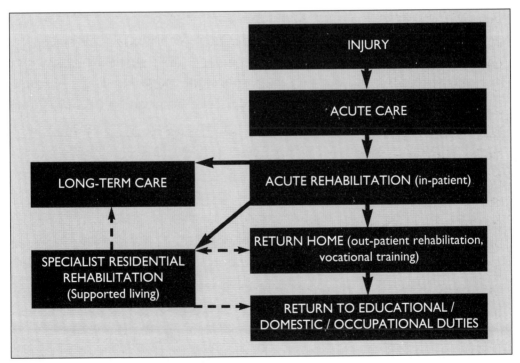

Figure 5 *The possibilities of care*

independent living with minimum or no supervison. The type of residential care depends on the level of dependency of the patient. It is hoped that patients move along a continuum from high dependency (hospital, nursing homes) to lower dependency (group home, sheltered accommodation) to independence, although not everyone will be able to achieve this.

The ultimate aim is for the person with the head injury to be reintegrated into the community from where they came. This means gradually and progressively taking on appropriate activities and responsibilities. It may mean vocational retraining, altering jobs and accepting early retirement from the workplace. The person has to build a new life and this takes a considerable time.

Learning From Carlos

Carlos was a thirty-eight-year-old minicab driver with a wife, Jenny, and seven-year-old son, John, when he had his accident. His severe head injury left him with an impaired memory, weak concentration, poor expressive and receptive speech, incontinence, a glass eye, agitation, restlessness, lowered tolerance, and both verbal and physical aggression. After three weeks at a regional rehabilitation centre, staff concluded that they could not manage his restlessness, wandering, verbal and physical abuse. He was transferred to a local psychiatric hospital where he remained as a resident on an acute admission ward for one year. Everybody agreed that Carlos was inappropriately placed on the psychiatric ward and his behaviour became increasingly difficult to manage. A nurse would usually have to sit at the door to stop Carlos escaping and when frustrated he would often become aggressive. Carlos had a negative effect on staff morale and it was noted that certain psychiatric patients were discharging themselves, saying they could not tolerate Carlos' constant restlessness and shouting. As the noise got louder, the pleas for something to be done went higher up the management chain of command, until money was made available for an assessment at a private rehabilitation unit which specialized in the behavioural treatment of challenging behaviour following brain injury.

Carlos' behaviour during the six-week assessment at the secure treatment unit was characterized by aggression, lack of co-operation and constant requests to be allowed to go home. At the end of this period, the ten professionals involved in his case unanimously agreed that Carlos needed to be admitted; it was felt that the unit's behaviour modification programme could help him improve his behaviour. Only Carlos was adamant that he did not want to stay there but wanted to go home. Jenny, with the child to look after, felt dreadfully torn between the voices of the professionals and that of her husband. To everybody's surprise she said, "I cannot leave him here if he doesn't want to stay. I will take him home if you can give me some help."

A community care package was put together which involved recruiting a private community psychiatric nurse, called Bob, who would work with Carlos during the day while Jenny was at work and John was at school; there would also be back-up from the local clinical psychologist. Nobody was sure how the programme would work.

Contrary to expectations the programme worked exceedingly well. Carlos' behaviour improved dramatically with his return home. Bob encouraged him to get dressed and shave, make cups of tea, wash and iron his clothes, cook and go to the shops. They also went out socially, visited places of interest, and embarked on decorating the house and gardening. After six months Carlos managed to cook a meal of lamb chops, potatoes and carrots. In the out-patient clinic when visiting the psychologist he was neat, appropriate and polite, hardly recognizable as the man who had terrorized a psychiatric ward.

After the programme had been running for eight months, Carlos decided that he did not need Bob any more and that he would rather be on his own. The professionals involved, and Jenny, were concerned as to whether this would be a good idea, but were forced into relinquishing Bob's services when Carlos locked him out of the house and refused to see him again. After one year, Carlos decided that he did not want to see the clinical psychologist any more, because he did not like the psychologist making appointments with Jenny behind his back. He explained that he was now the boss and was in control. If an appointment needed to be made, he would make it himself. This assertive behaviour on Carlos' part was unexpected, but it was also an indication of the dramatic progress towards independence that Carlos had made over the last 12 months.

The lessons to be learned from Carlos seem to be, firstly, always listen to the voice of the person with the head injury. Professionals and carers should be aware of getting left behind as the head-injured person moves from the position of being a dependent patient, where decisions are largely made for him, to an independent adult with impairments, who needs to feel in control and make his own decisions. Secondly, a well thought-out package of rehabilitative care, tailored to the needs of the person with the head injury, in the community where he lives, can often be as effective, and less expensive, than an institution-based programme. ■

ASSESSMENT

During all the stages of rehabilitation, and throughout the process of care, accurate assessment is vital. We all make everyday assessments of people's abilities with statements like, "He's very bright", "She's very caring" or "He's incompetent." After a serious head injury, the patient is left with an unknown mixture of physical, mental, emotional and behavioural strengths and weaknesses which the carers, the professionals and the patient himself need to assess and understand. The assessment and understanding is important for a number of reasons:

I   Once a problem is clearly identified it can be 'worked on' — new skills, compensatory strategies and aids can be used.

DATE

BOWELS
0 = incontinent
1 = occasional accident
2 = continent

BLADDER
0 = incontinent or catheterized and unable to manage
1 = occasional accident (max 1 x per 24 hours)
2 = continent (for over 7 days)

GROOMING
0 = needs help
1 = independent, face / hair /teeth / shaving

TOILET USE
0 = dependent
1 = needs some help, but can do something
2 = independent (on and off, dressing, wiping)

FEEDING
0 = unable
1 = needs help cutting, spreading butter etc
2 = independent

TRANSFER
0 = unable
1 = major help (1–2 people, physical)
2 = minor help (verbal or physical)
3 = independent

MOBILITY
0 = immobile
1 = wheelchair — independent, including corners etc
2 = walks with help of 1 person (verbal or physical)
3 = independent (but may use any aid, eg. stick)

DRESSING
0 = dependent
1 = needs help, but can do about half unaided
2 = independent

STAIRS
0 = unable
1 = needs help (verbal, physical, carrying aid)
2 = independent up and down

BATHING
0 = dependent
1 = independent

TOTAL

The index should be used as a record of what the patient *does*, not as a record of what he *could* do. The main aim is to establish the degree to which the patient is independent of any physical or verbal help.

Figure 6 *The Barthel Activities of Daily Living (ADL) Index* (adapted from Mahoney FI & Barthel DW, 'Functional evaluation: the Barthel index', *Maryland State Medical Journal* 14, pp 61-5, 1965)

2   Good assessment enables those involved to monitor progress. This feedback is important for giving direction, encouraging and motivating the patient. Very often the person with the head injury will not recognize the progress he has made and will constantly compare his abilities with those before the injury rather than immediately afterwards.

3   Assessment gives a clearer, more realistic picture and, it is hoped, helps to reduce anxiety. If you do not know what is wrong you can start imagining all sorts of things. People can sometimes blame themselves for difficulties, or feel guilty about things which are not their fault but are the direct result of the brain injury.

Formal assessments will be carried out by occupational therapists, a speech therapist, a clinical psychologist, physiotherapists and nurses.

A useful measure of basic self-care skills necessary for physical independence is the Barthel Activity of Daily Living Index (Figure 6). This scale is useful as it can measure changes in the early weeks and months after head injury and can be completed by relatives and carers. The measurement is on a 20 point scale where an unconscious patient would score nought throughout and a score of 20 would suggest physical independence. It is important to use the index as a record of what the patient does, not as a record of what he could do. So, for example, when scoring 'Bathing', the patient would score one if he independently managed to have a bath on his own, not if he had to be continually reminded, then prompted and helped. The main aim is to establish a degree of independence from any physical or verbal help.

STAGES OF RECOVERY

It is important to recognize that, following head injury, the pathway to recovery is divided into a number of recognized stages. Of course these stages are not set in stone; some people's experience may be quite different, or some may have a different array of symptoms and not recognize these stages. However, for a large number of individuals with severe head injury, these stages may be familiar. It is helpful to recognize the pathway so that you have a clear idea of where you are heading. It is also extremely important to treat the individuals according to their stage of recovery.

First Stage

The patient is in a coma and is very reliant on medical help. It is the family who must bear the emotional and psychological burden caused by the injury. The family deal with feelings of helplessness, denial, shock and confusion.

Second and Third Stages

The second stage is usually the one where the patient is coming out of a coma and into post-traumatic amnesia. It is characterized by either severe agitation, restlessness, confusion or a persistent vegetative state. In the third stage, if the patient is conscious, he will have severe attentional, problem-solving, social and memory deficits, but will often deny the reality of these problems. Rather he will be more likely to focus on and complain of physical injuries, particularly if orthopaedic injuries were sustained.

Fourth Stage

The patient is becoming increasingly aware of cognitive deficits in memory, attention, thinking and planning and difficulties with tiredness. This often leads to frustration, irritability, anger and the beginning of anxiety and depression. They may appear to be relatively normal and there may be some pressure to return to work or school, or household responsibilities. This may prove to be more difficult than initially imagined and may end in failure, increasing the patient's awareness of the real difficulties. It is usual for the patient to over-estimate his abilities and under-estimate the problems at this stage. There may also be some emotional lability and lowered tolerance of frustration.

After a head injury some people experience problems. Please go through the list and circle the number which is closest to how severe this particular problem is for you, your loved one or your acquaintance, compared with **how things were before the accident.**

0 = not experienced at all   3 = a moderate problem
1 = no longer a problem   4 = a severe problem
2 = a mild problem

		0	1	2	3	4
1	Difficulties in movement or mobility	0	1	2	3	4
2	Lack of strength in arms and hands	0	1	2	3	4
3	Loss of senses (smell, taste, touch, temperature)	0	1	2	3	4
4	Visual difficulties (restricted, double or blurred vision)	0	1	2	3	4
5	Hearing disturbances	0	1	2	3	4
6	Feelings of dizziness, loss of balance	0	1	2	3	4
7	Increased sensitivity to noise, light	0	1	2	3	4
8	Headaches — more frequent/severe	0	1	2	3	4
9	Tiring more easily — fatigue	0	1	2	3	4
10	Sleep disturbances	0	1	2	3	4
11	Epileptic seizures	0	1	2	3	4
12	Forgetfulness — poor memory	0	1	2	3	4
13	Poor concentration — easily distracted	0	1	2	3	4
14	Taking longer to think	0	1	2	3	4
15	Difficulty planning and organizing	0	1	2	3	4
16	Difficulty finding the right words — less fluent in conversation	0	1	2	3	4
17	Difficulty carrying out more than one task at a time	0	1	2	3	4
18	Difficulty reading, spelling or writing	0	1	2	3	4
19	Being more rigid — less flexible, in thinking and behaviour	0	1	2	3	4
20	Feeling tearful or depressed	0	1	2	3	4
21	Feeling worried or anxious	0	1	2	3	4
22	Lack of motivation, initiative and drive	0	1	2	3	4
23	Changes in emotions — either more or less emotional	0	1	2	3	4
24	Loss of confidence	0	1	2	3	4
25	Making inappropriate or insensitive comments or actions	0	1	2	3	4
26	Lack of awareness of changes in self (insight)	0	1	2	3	4
27	Being irritable — easily frustrated/quick to anger	0	1	2	3	4
28	Changes in level of sexual interest — either more or less	0	1	2	3	4
29	Maintaining previous workload/standard	0	1	2	3	4
30	Difficulties maintaining good relationships	0	1	2	3	4
31	Participating in previous leisure activities	0	1	2	3	4
32	Participating in previous social activities	0	1	2	3	4
33	Any other problems	0	1	2	3	4

Figure 7 *Problem checklist*

Fifth Stage

At this stage there is some improvement in general mental abilities, although the patient is still typically experiencing mild to moderate memory problems, problem-solving difficulties, mild word-finding difficulties and emotional difficulties. Very often his ability to cope in structured situations is good, but less good in unstructured or stressful situations. When presented with complex material he may become lost in detail and miss out on the main idea. It is with the improvements in mental abilities that the patient becomes more insightful, and aware of his disabilities and the realities of his new life. There is a tendency to refer back to 'his old self', rather than how he was immediately after his injury. These comparisons can lead to significant depression and anxiety as the individual begins to accept the losses and changes that have taken place in his life. This stage of beginning to come to terms emotionally with what has happened is often the most difficult for patients.

Sixth Stage

At this stage the person with the head injury is aware of his residual deficits and has come to accept them emotionally. The cognitive problems with memory, attention and problem solving are now less severe and the person has returned to taking on some of his old responsibilities. Individuals still become tired easily and 'overdo it', and then may exhibit some of the cognitive and emotional behaviour of stages four and five, but this becomes less frequent. The individual gradually takes on more of old responsibilities, rebuilding confidence and self-esteem and, it is hoped, building a new life for himself.

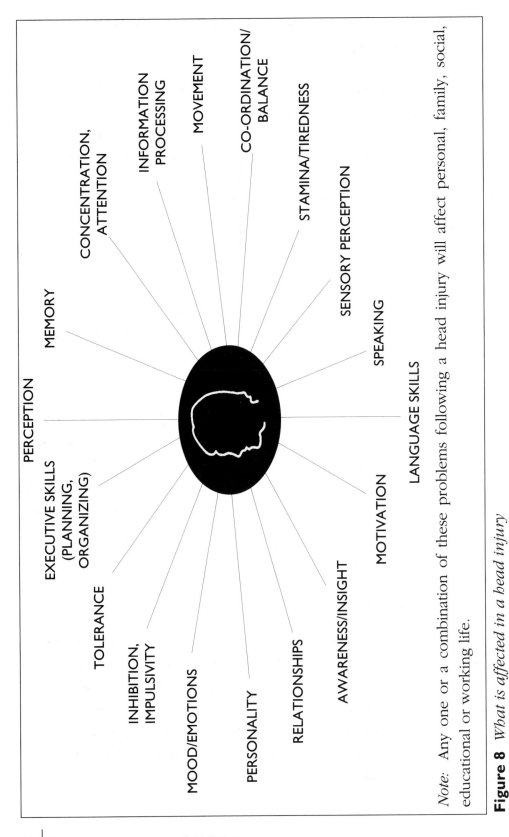

Note: Any one or a combination of these problems following a head injury will affect personal, family, social, educational or working life.

Figure 8 *What is affected in a head injury*

Encouraging Thoughts

1 A person who is severely impaired never knows his inner source of strength until he is treated like a real person.

2 Nothing equals the power of love. It's the only source of magic there is.

3 People who have had a head injury do not want hand-outs, but hand-ups.

4 Think positively about the gains made since the accident, rather than comparing with how things used to be before it.

5 What do you dream about? You can do anything, but you may have to do it differently.

Input from health service professionals is very high in the early stages when the problems are largely medical. As time goes by the problems alter and become largely social, psychological and environmental. These types of difficulty are more subtle, more difficult to observe and more difficult to overcome. However, a large proportion of people with head injuries reach stage six and can live a fulfilling, independent life with their disability.

Peeling Potatoes

"Two years after my son came out of hospital after a severe head injury, I remember standing at the sink peeling some potatoes for our tea. It suddenly struck me, 'Why am I doing this for him while he sits and watches TV?' I said, 'Come on Pat, you can have a go at this.' He did, with some reluctance at first, but I now see it as a turning-point, because I began to stop doing everything for him and he started doing things for himself." ■

IMPROVING EVERYDAY LIVING SKILLS

For most patients, everyday living skills, such as washing, dressing and carrying out domestic chores, return quite spontaneously, but for others it is a question of relearning those basic skills to remedy this deficit. The key to relearning a basic skill is to break it down into its smaller component parts. Any skill can be broken down into a number of set stages. Once these are listed, the patient is prompted verbally to carry out each individual stage. Once he can go through the individual stages, prompts can be grouped together so that the number of prompts gradually decreases, as in the following example, making a cup of tea.

Ten prompts	*Three prompts*
Fill kettle	
Turn on power	Boil kettle
Get cup	
Put tea bag in cup	
Put boiling water in cup	Prepare cup
Leave for one minute	
Remove tea bag	
Put milk in cup	Add milk, sugar
Put sugar in cup	
Stir it up	

It is a useful idea to write the list of instructions on a cue card and place it in a strategic position in an appropriate room. It is important to establish a routine and to make sure that all items are kept in their proper places. Life is difficult enough without having to hunt around to find where somebody else has put the tea bags. 'A place for everything and everything in its place' is also a useful cue card to have displayed on the wall in a prominent position.

Managing money can often be a problem and, like all other everyday skills, it may be of benefit to break down the larger task into smaller skills. Confidence and skill can be rebuilt by progressing from simple to complex tasks. Perhaps the first step might be buying one item from a shop, using coins, then moving up to notes, then checking change and then writing cheques. It is important to recognize difficulties and to accept the adage that small steps mean progress.

We often take for granted our ability to structure our day and manage our time. This can often be a problem if a person has been out of action while in hospital, or if a person has memory or organizational difficulties since receiving a head injury. Again it is helpful to start off by structuring the person's day with set activities, usually written down on a wall chart. It then becomes clear what needs to be done and also what has been done — providing information and feedback. Gradually the individual will take over more responsibility for establishing a schedule, as he relearns how to make decisions about the use of time. Once a routine has been established, the wall chart becomes less of a prompt, as the person becomes more independent.

UNDERSTANDING AND COPING WITH THE PHYSICAL EFFECTS OF HEAD INJURY

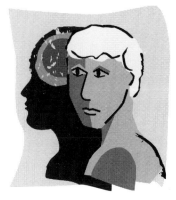

Chapter 4

Introduction

Around 90 per cent of people who have severe head injuries make what is known as an 'excellent physical recovery' by the end of the first year. This often means that there are no obvious visible physical disabilities such as difficulty walking or talking. However there may well be more subtle difficulties, such as excessive tiredness or headaches, which are not so apparent, but nevertheless can be a problem. Improvement in physical ability, involving movement, tends to come quite early on and has the advantage of being easily measured, making the patient more aware of progress. Research suggests that, although physical symptoms are a problem, they do not create as much distress for the patient, family or carers as cognitive, behavioural and emotional symptoms.

Movement, Co-ordination and Balance

Many people ask the question, "Why does a head injury affect my ability to walk or pick up a book? My muscles seem all right. I did not injure my arms or legs." To answer this question we need to consider the process involved in picking up a cup. The movement starts as a thought, "I'll pick that cup up", which then produces a mental programme, or sequence of actions, which occurs so rapidly that we are not aware of it. The thought and subsequent programme then produce a series of actions. The mental activity is largely centred around a particular part of the brain, known as the motor cortex (the area on the border between the frontal and parietal lobes, see Figure 2). From here a series of messages or nerve impulses travel down a long chain of relay stations: the message is passed to the brain stem, down the spinal cord to the nerve cells that link directly with the muscles concerned. This command makes sure that each necessary muscle is relaxed and contracted at the right moment. It is worth remembering that there are over 30 individual muscles in one arm. Damage to any part of this long pathway from brain to muscle will disturb motor control.

Damage to the brain that causes these types of movement difficulties usually happens to the motor cortex, the brain stem and the cerebellum (see Figure 9). When severe impairment in movement has occurred, it is often the case that a blood clot has pressurized and damaged the motor cortex. As one side of the brain affects the motor co-ordination of the opposite side of the body, the patient often experiences a weakness or paralysis of one side (hemiplegia or hemiparesis). So for example, if a blood clot pressurizes the right hemisphere motor cortex, one would expect the patient to have difficulty moving the left arm and leg.

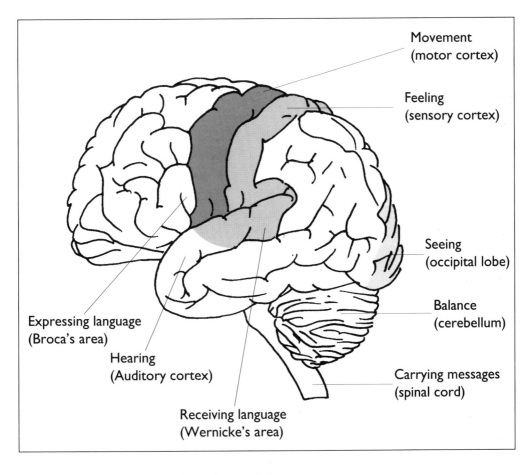

Figure 9 *The brain and its physical functions*

Damage to the cerebellum is known to affect the fine co-ordination of muscles, leading to strong but clumsy movements. This means that it is difficult to stand, to walk steadily or to balance, for example to carry a cup of tea without spilling it. As recovery begins and movement returns, physical ability comes back, but it is still difficult to co-ordinate finely tuned, skilful jobs requiring dexterity, such as threading needles. Cerebellar inco-ordination is difficult to treat. The emphasis is on practising weight-bearing activities. Weighted aids such as shoes or wrist bands can have some effect in reducing and steadying tremors.

Difficulties with balance can be created by damage to the 'vestibular system', which is a small delicate piece of equipment enclosed in a dense bone at the back of the skull. Even mild head injury can upset this delicate organ, so that the person often feels dizzy or as if his head is starting to spin with a sudden movement.

In the early days after a head injury, while the patient is lying in bed, the legs and arms may be stiff and straight. It is important to move these limbs regularly, so that contractures do not develop later on. A contracture is defined as the 'abnormal shortening of muscle tissue, rendering the muscle highly resistant to stretching'. If the muscle or joint is not exercised but stays in the same position it will shorten and lose its ability to stretch, or contract and relax. At this early stage the physiotherapist will be involved in providing an exercise programme. Less severe contractures will normally respond quite quickly to a dynamic programme of learning new movements. At a later stage, more severe contractures may require the muscle to be stretched, then encased in plaster. After a few days the plaster may be cut and 'wedged' further in order to produce more stretch on the contracted joint.

In order for a person to regain normal movement, they will have to relearn the basic developmental stages or sequences. In the same way that babies cannot run before they can walk, or walk before they can balance, the patient needs to get the basic stages in the correct order first. If he gets one stage wrong, all subsequent stages will be wrong. For example, balance in standing is needed before walking, stability of shoulders comes before hands can be brought together in the mid-line, and head control is needed before eyes can focus. Abnormal posture due to contractures or spasticity will, by necessity, result in abnormal movement. If that abnormal movement is constantly produced, it becomes reinforced as a habit and becomes an automatically learned response. The essential task is therefore to get the building-blocks of movement right to start off with and build on from there.

The physiotherapist is the key professional at this stage, who will demonstrate and then help the patient practise these movements and postures. Depending on the patient's ability, exercises may be carried out on a mat, an inflatable mattress, in a pool or on parallel bars. Endurance and strength need to be gradually built up. The patient will inevitably have a tendency to over-use his good limbs. This is understandable as early attempts to use a paralysed limb may be unsuccessful, so the brain automatically learns not to use it. This tendency needs to be overcome deliberately, otherwise progress will be limited. The slightest movement in the paralysed limb should be encouraged, with the use of the good one being progressively restricted at the same time. In this way the patient will be forced to use the affected part.

DYSPRAXIA

Dyspraxia is a disorder of deliberate voluntary actions, or sequences of action, that is, it is different from problems with motor co-ordination or movement. The patient may not have a problem with actual movement, rather the problem lies with being unable to put movements together deliberately and intentionally. For example, if the patient is asked to bend his elbow he may not be able to do it, but five minutes later, if he is asked to look at his watch, he may bend his elbow quite automatically. The problem lies with the patient's inability to conceptualize, initiate and perform the sequence. He may not be able to repeat gestures such as saluting, deliberately touching his index finger to his thumb, tapping or, more importantly, getting dressed, putting his trousers on or tying a tie. The patient may say,

"I know what to do but I can't do it." These sorts of difficulties can often be misunderstood by relatives and carers, who wrongly interpret this behaviour as a lack of co-operation.

Paul: The Lionheart

Paul was involved in a motor-cycle accident when he was 19 years old. He was always something of a loner, a rebel who kicked against authority, after a difficult childhood when his parents separated. He suffered a severe head injury which left him with physical, mental, emotional and speech problems. He wore thick glasses which were patched over one eye, he was restricted to a wheelchair, his speech was slurred and his memory and concentration were appalling. He was a dreadful patient, abusive to physiotherapists, occupational therapists and nurses. He would knock things over on the ward, hit people, swear and sulk. He was labelled a 'behavioural problem' by those who did not know or understand him. The only place Paul felt safe and happy was the local Headway House, where he became very attached to the motherly co-ordinator. When people got to know Paul they realized that the label 'behavioural problem' was totally misleading. He was a tough guy on the outside, but inside, a real softy. He had a single-minded determination that he would walk again, but he had severe ataxia, co-ordination problems and paralysis. He pushed himself, spending a great deal of time in the multi-gym strengthening his muscles. He gradually progressed from wheelchair, to frame, to sticks. After four years of attending Headway he acquired a place in a special village for disabled people. He knew it was a step forward, and accepted the placement with gritted teeth as he knew he would desperately miss the warmth and comfort of the Headway centre. Almost 10 years after his injury he returned to the Headway centre, staggering with arms and legs flying, his 13 stone of solid muscle miraculously keeping him balanced. "You see, no sticks. I told you I'd walk eventually." ■

Rehabilitative treatment aims at breaking tasks down into set sequences of activities, and then practising each stage in the sequence. Initially, with the help of the therapist, the patient has to repeat one sequence constantly, with physical, verbal or visual cues, such as an instruction board. When the patient gets better at the sequences, the verbal and visual prompts are reduced and gradually withdrawn.

LOSS OF SENSATION

Just as a part of the brain deals with movement, there is also a part that specifically deals with processing information about the sensations of sight, hearing, smell, taste and touch. After head injury, people may lose some of the different senses, but the actual sense organs themselves, that is the eyes, ears, nose, tongue and skin, are not damaged. This is again because the damage is in the area of central processing rather than at the level of the sensory organ itself. There is a part of the cerebrum called the sensory cortex (see Figure 9). If this has been damaged by bruising or squashing it is put out of action for a while, although often there is gradual recovery after a few weeks or months. If this area has been torn, it is unlikely to return to normal functioning. Different parts of the sensory cortex deal with the sensations experienced in different parts of the body. Sensation can be tested by touching different areas of the body with cotton wool for light touch, and a blunt object such as a pencil for deep sensation.

Similarly visual problems are often not the result of damage to the eyes, but to the parts of the brain that interpret and process what the eyes actually see. This might result in problems with judging distances, having blurred or double vision, or neglecting to notice part of the visual field. Processing what the eyes see is carried out right at the back of the brain in the occipital lobe. If the occipital lobes are severely damaged the patient may be blinded, or if either the right or left occipital lobe is damaged, problems may occur in one aspect of his visual field. In this case a person may walk into doors, misjudge distances, ignore the print on one side of a

Using Aids

There are a number of companies producing rehabilitation aids which can make life easier. Your local occupational therapist should also be able to advise on where to buy the following aids. It is important not to introduce aids too early, or more than one at a time, as they can reduce motivation and stop the patient reaching their full potential. The following list provides just a few examples of the type of aids available:

Dressing   Special latch hook buttons (as used in rug making) can be useful. Elasticated cuffs on shirts and blouses help avoid difficult extra buttons. Front-fastening bras or adapted Velcro fastenings can make an awkward task easier. For shoes choose trainers with Velcro fastenings and slip-on styles.

Eating   Plates with a raised edge to prevent the food from spilling are available in a number of designs; also flat surrounds which can be attached to a normal plate. Specially available non-slip place mats prevent plates and dishes slipping around during use. Other plates or bowls can be attached to a large suction device for greater anchorage. There is special cutlery such as the Rocker and Nelson knives, Splayds or Sporks, which are also handy.

Food preparation   There is a variety of one-handed, electric or wall-mounted tin-openers which can make life easier. Similarly there is a variety of special jar- and bottle-openers which enable a person to grip an object by pushing their body against the clamp, leaving the hands free to remove a lid. Food processors and microwave ovens are invaluable. Putting vegetables into a mesh chip basket inside a saucepan avoids the need to carry hot saucepans full of boiling water around the kitchen.

Housework   Washing up and ironing are very difficult to do with one hand. If affordable, it is a good idea to buy a dishwasher and tumble drier.

piece of paper or only shave half his face, put on only one sock, shoe or glove, or eat the food off one side of the plate. This area will be covered in more detail under perceptual problems (page 86). Temperature control can also be adversely affected, particularly by damage to the brain stem. The person with a head injury may feel very hot, even on a cold day, or vice versa. These inbuilt bodily thermostats seem to become faulty particularly when the person is feeling tired.

TIREDNESS

Tiredness, loss of stamina and fatigue after head injury are some of the most limiting residual symptoms because they affect everything that the person does. The problem is that the person tires more quickly and more extremely. Patients often say, "It is a little like when you are driving your car and you run out of petrol — very suddenly there is no energy in the tank and you have to stop." The reason for this type of difficulty is probably that the part of the brain, the brain stem, which controls consciousness, wakefulness and the rhythm of sleeping has been damaged. Difficulties are often exacerbated if the person with the head injury does not accept that this is a problem and thinks, "I've just got to keep pushing myself." If you have been used to driving a car with a 12-gallon petrol tank and suddenly change to one with an eight-gallon tank, no amount of pushing is going to make up for that lost capacity. Similar problems can be created if the person denies that they are tired, because they may become moody, agitated or withdrawn instead.

A person with a head injury complaining of tiredness probably actually is tired. If they really overdo it and deplete their store of energy, it may take all of the next day to catch up and replenish that store or refill the tank. The best way for the person with a head injury to manage this problem is to:

(a) recognize early signs of fatigue and take it easy;

(b) carefully plan activities to avoid doing too much;

(c) be aware of well meaning associates who do not understand the problem and encourage the patient to do too much;

(d) plan adequate periods of rest, especially after tiring activities;

(e) remember that eating a meal can sometimes help.

Someone with a head injury should not be too proud to go to bed and sleep for an hour in the afternoon.

HEADACHE

Up to 25 per cent of people who have suffered a severe head injury still suffer from headaches two years after the injury. These are unlike normal headaches in their intensity, duration and frequency. The effects range from mild, occasional inconvenience to nearly total incapacitation. These headaches are generally aggravated by stress, tension, or by the patient trying to 'do too much', and can be helped by a stress management programme, the same medication as used for migraine treatment, muscle relaxation exercises or acupuncture.

SPEAKING AND SWALLOWING DISORDERS

The muscles in our mouths do not seem very important unless we are, for example, brushing our teeth, pulling a funny face or putting on lipstick, but they can be severely affected by a head injury, particularly if there is damage to a cranial nerve. The muscles needed for articulation of speech thereby become weak and unco-ordinated. This condition, known as 'dysarthria', may cause speech to be extremely slurred, slower, or quieter than normal, making it hard for others to understand. The speech therapist can help the patient in relearning basic muscle movements and improving quality of speech, at least to a limited degree.

A person whose head injury has damaged their ability to chew and swallow is said to have 'dysphagia'. If this condition is too severe it may result in malnutrition, or problems with food falling into the airway, which can result in illness or choking. In some cases it may be safest for the patient to be fed through a nasogastric tube or gastrostomy, at least in the short term. Again the speech therapist is the key professional involved in helping the patient to improve these vital functions.

EPILEPSY

Injury to the surface of the brain, in the form of a scar, increases the risk of an epileptic attack. This is more likely to happen in the case of penetrating injuries, where the skull has been fractured and a piece of bone, or something else, has penetrated the brain. Although the wound heals, the resulting scar causes the electrical activity in that area to be unstable and liable to bursts of uncontrollable activity.

Epileptic fits or seizures vary in severity from 'grand mal' seizures where the electrical activity affects the whole brain, to 'petit mal' or focal seizures where the electrical disturbance remains localized to a small area. 'Grand mal' seizures involve widespread muscle contraction, rapid body movement, sometimes loss of bladder and bowel control, irregular breathing and loss of consciousness. There is usually little or no warning, although some patients know when they are going to have a seizure by having a feeling beforehand which is called an 'aura', often involving a full feeling in the pit of the stomach that moves up towards the mouth. Partial or focal seizures are very different and may only involve a lapse of concentration, losing the thread of what was being said, a twitch of a little finger or performing a repetitive task such as picking at their clothes.

These seizures frequently arise from scar tissue around the temporal lobes and are often difficult to diagnose.

One person in every hundred of the general population suffers from epilepsy, though few have head injuries. Seizures occur in 35 per cent of patients with 'open or penetrating head injuries'. Although most seizures occur within the first week after an injury, the first may not occur until one to two years after. A patient may not be considered free of symptoms until two or three seizure-free years have passed. Even then, there is a 5 per

---

What to Do About an Epileptic Fit

If you have had a head injury and are liable to attacks, you may be able to recognize the warning signs and to sit down and tell somebody what is going to happen. If you see somebody having a major fit, the first thing to do is to protect the person from hurting themselves and to prevent unnecessary anxiety in others.

- Be calm — talk to them gently and calmly.

- Make sure the person is able to breathe freely: loosen clothing and buttons around the neck.

- Do not place anything in the mouth, as it is likely to cause more harm than good.

- The person having the fit should be placed on their side, with something soft beneath the head, and only moved if they are in a dangerous position.

- On recovery there may be a temporary period of confusion or headache; the person should sit or lie quietly until this improves and be allowed to sleep, if they wish to do so.

---

cent chance that another seizure will occur in the future. For patients with 'closed' head injury there is only a 1 per cent chance of developing seizures. In the UK, if the patient has had an epileptic seizure, he is normally requested to surrender his driving licence. The licence is returned on medical advice, usually if the patient has been free of seizures for a period of two years.

Anybody can have a seizure, although this possibility may be increased by hunger (low blood sugar), exhaustion, over-breathing, anxiety and stress, alcohol and certain drugs. The likelihood of an attack is reduced by anticonvulsant medication such as sodium valproate (Epilim) and carbamazipine (Tegretol). The electrical activity of the brain can be measured by an EEG. This useful diagnostic tool is helpful in locating the cause of the seizure and providing evidence of abnormal activity, which might mean continuing on a course of anticonvulsant medication.

BLADDER AND BOWEL INCONTINENCE

After head injury a number of basic skills fall apart – skills which we have learnt as children but take for granted as adults, for example walking, writing and cooking. This unfortunately is also true of bladder and bowel control. It is actually a complicated skill: we have to detect the subtle, physical signs that we need to go to the toilet and then act on these signs. It is both a physical and a cognitive skill.

If incontinence is prolonged, patients are usually catheterized, which involves placing a tube in the bladder. When the catheter is removed, the patient should be given a regular programme where he is taken to the toilet initially at least every two hours and twice at night. This interval is gradually prolonged until he has relearned the skill of picking up the early messages and signs and getting himself to the toilet. If incontinence continues, a detailed medical and behavioural assessment needs to be carried out. Factors such as medication, physical ability, communication problems, poor attention, the patient's ability physically to get to the toilet and embarrassment all need to be taken into account.

There are times when simply altering the patient's physical environment can affect incontinence. It may be that he has difficulty getting to the toilet in time, or that the physical effort involved may be so great that he prefers to wet or soil himself. In these situations the carer needs to ensure that the patient's bedroom is near the toilet and that the door is well marked, or that he has a urine bottle or commode available. Remember that coffee, tea, alcohol and some soft drinks have a diuretic effect and are bladder irritants, which may be adding to the problem.

At times a patient may be incontinent either as a way of getting attention or as a way of objecting to treatment. A simple behaviour modification programme may help. The first step is to keep a careful record of when, where and how often wetting or soiling occurs. Look for patterns such as which nursing staff were on, or how the patient was feeling. Once this record has been kept you then have a baseline of the frequency of the event. Then change the consequences or 'pay-offs' of the behaviour. Attention, praise or some other reward can be given for reducing the frequency of the incontinence. The 'structure' of the programme can help the patient feel more in control — they have a target to aim for. For more complex problems in this area, a clinical psychologist can be consulted.

UNDERSTANDING AND COPING WITH COGNITIVE SYMPTOMS AFTER HEAD INJURY

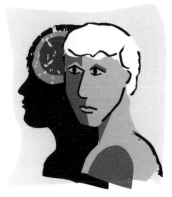

Chapter 5

INTRODUCTION

The word 'cognitive' refers to mental abilities such as speed of thought, memory, understanding, concentration, solving problems and using language. We are all blessed with these abilities to a greater or lesser extent. Recent research tells us that these different skills are all located in different areas of the brain and, although they are interrelated, they are also separate. We can think of our cognitive system as working in much the same way as a very advanced hi-fi system, which comes as a total package but is made up of a variety of individual parts. Some parts are more central than others. The whole system will fail to work if there is no power but if the amplifier is faulty the other areas may well light up although not producing any sound. On the other hand, if the record deck is damaged, this should not affect the smooth running of the radio, cassette deck or CD player. The human cognitive system is similarly complex.

A head injury is the equivalent of shaking up this very complex, delicate hi-fi system; some parts will be damaged, other parts may work perfectly well. It is important to understand which parts are working and which parts are faulty. In this chapter, the cognitive system has been conveniently, and rather simply, divided into six component parts: (1) memory; (2) attention or concentration; (3) speed of information processing; (4) executive functioning, or planning and organizing; (5) visuo-spatial and perceptual processing; and (6) language skills. For each component we will, firstly, look at everyday examples of what happens when there is a breakdown in functioning; secondly, examine how these processes actually work; and, thirdly, examine strategies for improving these areas of functioning. The strategies and exercises are specifically designed for the person with the head injury, although they are applicable to anybody and everybody. We could all improve our memory, concentration or any of the other areas.

MEMORY

Different Types of Memory

The study of human memory has produced a vast library of theories, research and knowledge. In our analogy of the hi-fi system, memory is perhaps most closely represented by the cassette recorder. We will need to stretch this analogy and imagine that this recorder is so advanced that it has a special microphone and camera which can record sounds, pictures, smells, tastes, touch and emotions. Not only that, but attached to the recorder is a huge store or filing system full of prerecorded cassettes and tapes. Scientists generally believe that there are three stages of memory, which correspond to the microphone, the cassette recorder and the storage cabinet. These three stages of memory are called immediate or sensory memory, short-term or everyday memory, and long-term memory (Figure 10).

Our memory systems work initially by taking in information through our senses (sight, hearing, taste, smell, touch). This information goes into immediate or sensory memory, where it is held for a very brief period of time, usually a few seconds. The information is then passed on to short-term memory, where it is held for a short period and then rejected or passed on to long-term store. Information in the middle stage or short-term memory is a little like having a tape of a particular event on the tape deck: the information is recorded but will be erased, or taped over, unless that tape is taken out of the recording area and transferred to long-term store or the filing cabinet. Once that tape is in long-term store it is relatively safe, as long as you know where you have put it. The tapes in long-term store consist of memories of personal experiences, memories of all the knowledge and information we have learned, and memories for skills such as swimming or riding a bicycle.

Memory Problems Caused by Head Injury

The situation is further confused because there are a number of different types of memory problem normally associated with head injury (see

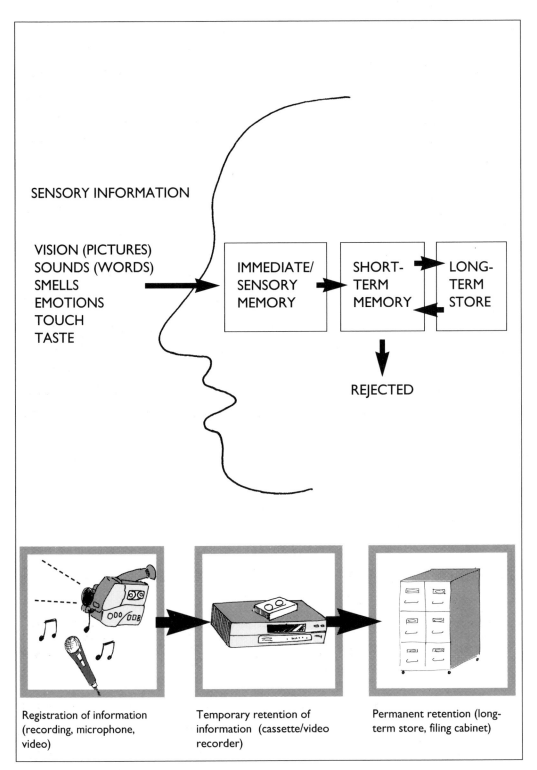

SENSORY INFORMATION

VISION (PICTURES)
SOUNDS (WORDS)
SMELLS
EMOTIONS
TOUCH
TASTE

IMMEDIATE/
SENSORY
MEMORY

SHORT-
TERM
MEMORY

LONG-
TERM
STORE

REJECTED

Registration of information (recording, microphone, video)

Temporary retention of information (cassette/video recorder)

Permanent retention (long-term store, filing cabinet)

Figure 10 *The three stages of memory*

Figure 11). First, there is post-traumatic amnesia (PTA), which we have already discussed in Chapter 2. This is the temporary state, immediately after the injury, where the patient is conscious, and appears relatively normal, but everyday memory is not working at all. The patient may have visitors and forget the visit 20 minutes later, may not be able to remember what day or time it is, or what was for breakfast that morning. In our hi-fi analogy, information is being recorded, but not being stored; the tape is being constantly played over rather than being taken out of the machine and stored in the filing cabinet. At a later date the patient will have no recollection of their time spent in PTA. For most people, problems associated with PTA are not important and quickly forgotten.

A second type of memory problem is termed 'retrograde amnesia'. This refers to the experience when the patient cannot remember personal information and events from the time period immediately preceding the accident and the accident itself. This form of memory loss stretches backwards from the accident for minutes, hours, days, months or sometimes years. For some people these memories come back gradually, or in patches, but for others there is a dense and permanent loss of

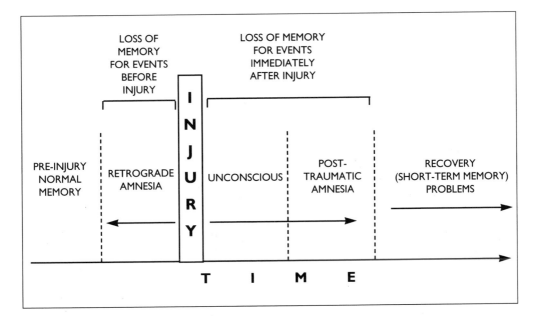

Figure 11 *Memory problems caused by head injury, related to time*

Retrograde Amnesia

Retrograde amnesia is loss of memory for events before the injury. Not being able to remember the injury, or the time immediately before, or a large chunk of one's past life, can create unusual problems, as our three examples demonstrate:

"I wish I could remember more about the accident. I am told that I was involved in a terrible crash on the motorway. It's like something that hasn't really happened to me. I can't remember the months before, or any pain, or being in hospital. It's like somebody else's story or a dream. I might as well have fallen out of an apple tree. It doesn't emotionally affect me. I want to remember what happened, what feelings I went through."

"I was 25 when I had my accident and could not remember anything from the previous year, including getting married to my wife. We therefore arranged to do it all over again and so had a second wedding ceremony."

"After being assaulted outside a public house I was left with a severe retrograde amnesia of some 15 years. This created enormous domestic problems as I could not remember my second wife, whom I had married two years ago, and who had lovingly nursed me back to health after my injury. However I had a very clear memory of my first wife, our wedding day and our happy marriage. I could not remember the bad last few years of my first marriage, where I am told our relationship turned sour and we argued and fought. I only have good memories and very positive feelings towards my first wife — I still love her — but unfortunately these feelings are not reciprocated."

memory. Retrograde amnesia is the equivalent of losing a cabinet full of prerecorded tapes of events and personal experiences.

The third and most common and troublesome form of memory problem is that commonly referred to as a problem of short-term memory, or 'everyday memory'. This type of problem means that the person with the head injury has difficulty remembering new facts, names, faces, appointments, where they have put things and what they have to do. Such problems disrupt all aspects of life, from work to social and leisure activities. Memory functioning is thought to be associated with the temporal lobe area of the brain. It is also thought that for most people the left temporal lobe is predominantly concerned with verbal memory and the right temporal lobe is predominantly associated with non-verbal, spatial, pictorial memory. There are no magic answers or wonder drugs to improve this type of memory problem, although there is often slow, gradual improvement over the years following the accident. The aims of rehabilitation are to help the person with a head injury improve his ability to cope with a poor memory by using a combination of external and internal strategies. Improvement comes with practising using recall strategies, not by simply practising random exercises. Memory is not like a muscle that can be developed purely by stretching it.

Examples of Short-term Memory Problems

1 "I constantly forget people's names."

2 "I forget where I put things and spend ages trying to find them."

3 "I often forget appointments or things I'm supposed to do."

4 "I just can't seem to grasp how to use that computer. One minute I think I've cracked it, but the next day I've forgotten the instructions."

5 "I walk into a room and forget what I was going to do."

Ways of Improving Your Memory

External strategies — using simple aids

Diary A diary is an essential adjunct to anybody's memory, whether for forward planning or for remembering past events. A page a day diary is most useful, so that you can write in appointments and also write down brief details of what you have done each day. These act as cues or triggers and mean that in future you will be able to remember a happy day or successful achievement. A small, portable dictaphone can also be useful.

Wall calendar/planner Keep a large wall calendar with enough room to write down important appointments and activities.

Labelling Label household items such as drawers or cupboards, jars of coffee or tea, rooms such as toilet or bathroom.

Lists Get into the habit of writing 'to do' lists for each day. Write down a list of instructions for using a computer or video and display it on the wall. Use shopping lists.

Positioning Become more organized at home — 'a place for everything and everything in its place'. Have a filing system for bills and letters. Position items where you are likely to remember them. Always put down an umbrella, briefcase or bag in front of you rather than beside or behind you. One person always kept the medication next to the milk in the fridge so that every morning when he had cereal for breakfast he remembered to take it. You can also buy specially designed pill boxes with separate compartments for days of the week.

Notes/signs Put a note or sign on the front door saying, 'Check to see if you've got everything.' Carry a small notebook or tear-off 'stickies'.

Watches/alarms A digital watch with an hourly bleep can remind the wearer of the passage of time or a special event. Alarms or bleepers on cookers or microwaves draw attention to the fact that the meal is cooked.

Internal strategies for improving memory

Repeat If you are trying to remember the name of somebody you have just met, repeat it to yourself under your breath, or even better, make a point of deliberately repeating their name back to them in conversation eg. 'right, John'.

Create an association Try to create an association with the name by relating it to a similar person you already know — think whether you like the name or not — or link it to a characteristic eg. Sandra has sandy-coloured hair.

Create a visual image It is said that 'a picture is worth a thousand words'. If you can create a visual picture out of a name you will have twice the chance of remembering it. For example, Mr Unwin could be pictured as an onion, or Mr Cohen could be visualized as having a head like an ice-cream cone or Mark could be visualized as having a big black mark across the line of his eyebrows. The more bizarre and exaggerated your image is, the easier it will be to remember, especially if it is linked to a physical characteristic of the person. By creating a visual image you are using the right side of your brain as well as the left side, so you will have twice the chance of remembering it.

Learning cues Most people can only remember six to seven things at the same time. So, if you have read a dense informative article, just list six points to remember, then reduce those six points to six key words. Those six key words will act as cues to gain access to the large body of information in the article. Maximum learning will be achieved by gradually lengthening the gap between rehearsing those cues — rehearse them after a five-minute gap, then an hour, then the next day.

Problem solving Trace your movements back step by step — if you have misplaced a key or wallet trace your steps back. Ask yourself, "Where would I put that key now?" When trying to recall a name think of the situation where you first met the person and learned their name.

George's Memory

"I do carry a diary and note book, have a wall calendar and planner which certainly help, but occasionally, when the unexpected happens, my memory gets me into trouble.

The worst incident occurred a while ago when I went shopping to a department store with the specific intention of buying a new jacket. On the way to the jacket section, I passed the shoe department and thought I'd try a pair on because they sell extra large shoes which fit my feet. After I'd tried the shoes on, I noticed an old friend over by the jackets and walked over to talk to him. We both tried on a number of different jackets as we talked, but neither of us liked any. His wife then arrived and they left together. As I couldn't find a jacket I liked, I left the store a couple of minutes later, deliberately thinking, 'I went in to buy a jacket — nothing else — I haven't forgotten anything have I?' Twenty yards down the high street, I heard a security man behind me shouting at somebody. To my surprise and embarrassment I realized it was me. I had forgotten to take the new shoes off! I laughed but the security man did not think that it was funny and I was taken to the police station. I told the police doctor about my head injury and memory problems, but even he did not fully believe me. I got very angry with him and ended up being charged and having to attend the local magistrates court.

Thankfully, I can laugh about the incident now — you have to. The key to the situation was that I was distracted. First by the temptation to try the shoes on, then by seeing my friend over on the other side of the store. It's like a train being derailed and ending up on the wrong track. I'm fine if I've just got one thing to do with no distractions, then I can keep on the right track." ■

ATTENTION AND CONCENTRATION

Examples of Attentional Difficulties

1   "I find it difficult to do more than one thing at a time, such as writing a message while answering the telephone."

2   "My mind wanders while reading or watching television."

3   "I find it difficult to sustain a conversation if there are other people talking, or other noises in the background."

4   "I start to do something and get distracted into doing something different."

5   "I lose track of what I wanted to say in the middle of speaking."

Understanding Attentional Difficulties

The ability to attend and concentrate comprises a number of stages of mental skill. We have to select something to concentrate on; we then have to ignore or filter out all other distractions; we have to maintain that state of alertness and concentration, and then be able to shift our concentration when appropriate. These abilities are a prerequisite for independent living, working, learning of new skills and even social relationships. It is very common for this group of skills to be impaired following head injury as they are predominantly associated with the often damaged frontal lobe area of the brain.

Research has shown that people with a head injury have great difficulty doing two or more things simultaneously. If a person with a head injury is given a task such as to track a moving object on a screen, they do it just as well as anybody else, but, if you instruct them to track the moving object and repeat a string of numbers, they perform much worse than anybody else. It is as though the brain has gone back to a stage of development more noticeable in childhood. If you ask a two-year-old child to chew a toffee, walk and carry a cup at the same time they usually fail because they are not very good at doing more than one thing at a time.

Attentional problems are made much worse when the person is tired: the more tired we are, the more easily distracted. Stress and worry can also adversely affect attention. If we are thinking, "I can't do it", "I'll make a fool of myself", then attention will be diminished. A vicious circle is set up where stress leads to poor attention, which leads to more worry and stress, which leads to poorer attention. These types of difficulties are more likely to show up during unstructured tasks, where there is more opportunity for the mind to wander.

Coping with Attentional Difficulties

1   Set increasingly difficult tasks and targets to work towards. For example, play 'Snap', 'Dominoes', 'Connect Four', read a book or watch television for five minutes, then gradually increase the time on the task to 10 minutes. Make sure the task is not too difficult to start off with. Keep a record of progress and also include incentives and rewards, such as a present if you achieve a certain goal. Use a timer or an alarm watch to focus attention for a specific period.

2   Organize the environment to eliminate background noise and distractions, such as radios or people talking.

3   Place a 'picture' or 'cue card' in an obvious place to remind yourself to pay attention. It might read, 'What should I be doing now?' or 'Am I wandering?'

4   Know your own limitations. Try for something that is a little difficult but not too difficult, just out of grasp but not out of reach.

5   Develop strategies for dealing with emotional or stimulation overload. For example, if somebody is talking too quickly don't be embarrassed to say, "Excuse me, I think I've lost you. Could you repeat that slowly?"

Speed of Information Processing

Examples of Information-processing Difficulties

1 "It takes me much longer to answer questions. If my wife says, 'Do you want some more potatoes?' there is a pause while I think of what the question means before I put forward my answer. "

2 "If somebody tries to explain to me how to do a simple task on the computer, I have to tell them to slow down and repeat it a number of times before it sinks in. Before my accident I'd pick up instructions straight away."

3 "I used to be able to add up lists of figures in my head very quickly. Now it takes ages."

4 "If people talk very quickly I cannot take in and understand what they are saying."

5 "I used to be known as being quick-witted and always had a smart answer for everyone. Now I'm much slower and will often think of a funny comment five minutes after the conversation has ended."

Understanding Information-processing Difficulties

The speed with which the brain processes information is obviously interrelated to a number of other areas such as our ability to concentrate and our level of consciousness, but, in simple terms, this area of skill is concerned with how fast we can take in, process and act upon information or, in everyday language, 'how fast the cogs turn'. In the field of computer technology, modern computers take in information, process it and act on it with a relatively brief delay, whereas older models whirl and click while processing the information. After a head injury the brain slows down, reverting to the style of the older computer. This slowing down of mental efficiency is often due to 'diffuse axonal damage', meaning the whole of the brain has been shaken up, and the previous efficient transmissions between individual nerve cells, along millions of different pathways, no longer run as smoothly and efficiently.

Improving Speed of Information Processing

1   Try to keep mentally stimulated but make sure it is the right level of stimulation, not too little and not too much. If there is too much stimulation the brain will just cut it all out. Stimulation is anything that makes a person think and respond. It means a part of the brain is working; chemicals are being passed along those neural pathways. Passively watching television is not as stimulating as talking, playing a game or a puzzle, or doing a mathematical task, all of which actively make a demand on the brain.

2   The type of stimulation is important. Practise doing things that are difficult rather than easy and progressively set more difficult targets to achieve.

Executive Functioning (Planning, Organizing and Problem Solving)

Examples of Difficulties in Executive Functioning

1   "Since his head injury, my husband has difficulty understanding anything subtle or abstract that is not very straightforward or concrete. I said to him recently, 'You've got a very one-eyed view of this', and I had to explain exactly what I meant. His thinking has become very rigid and dogmatic. Once he gets an idea into his head, it's difficult to shift it."

2   "I used to be the marketing manager of a large computer company. My desk was a busy crossroads where information from the sales department, production and market research would meet. My specialist skill was to analyse all that information and decide what products we would 'push' next year. My desk was never cluttered. I'd move things in and out very quickly. After the accident I just couldn't do it — piles of paper built up until I was completely snowed under. I just couldn't pull it all together. I was made redundant last year."

3   "I used to be a skilled labourer erecting and finishing off partition walling. The process of finishing required a number of stages such as joining, priming, plastering, sanding, replastering, treating and painting. After my accident, I had great difficulty getting myself organized and keeping to the right sequence."

4   Bill has great difficulty learning from his mistakes. His manager had already thrown him out of his office and slammed the door in his face, but Bill kept knocking on the door. He seems to lack judgement and the subtle appreciation of when to hold back, and does not seem to 'profit from experience'.

5 "It took me all day to put a shelf up, whereas before the accident I'd have done it automatically in about 30 minutes. I really did have to sit down and plan and organize what I needed, then plan the stages involved, and what to do."

Understanding Executive Difficulties

The term 'executive function' describes a collection of skills which typify a good administrative executive. The executive is the person who needs to make long-term plans and goals, to organize steps to achieve those plans, to initiate, monitor and subtly adjust those plans when necessary and to have good judgement. He needs to know the sales figures, to organize the pension fund and to predict the future. The executive needs to be able to stand back and make an appraisal — to be able to 'see the wood from the trees'. This requires a particular type of flexible thinking, being able to think creatively (divergently), and also to be able to focus on details (think convergently). These types of thinking, planning and organizing skills are understood to be located in the frontal lobes of the brain. Damage to these areas often produces these subtle deficits recently labelled the 'Dysexecutive Syndrome'.

People with these executive deficits may perform very well on structured tests or work activities, where they know what they have to do: the task is very straightforward or concrete and is right in front of their noses. But in a less straightforward, unstructured situation that requires planning, organization and initiation, they have great difficulties.

Many people with these types of problems are not aware of the fact. They lack the ability to stand back and identify their own strengths and weaknesses, to be able to see things from another person's point of view, to be able to monitor and evaluate their behaviour or to be able to set realistic goals. This failure to self-correct or change behaviour often leads to failure in the work setting. Some improvement can be made in these executive skills if the person is aware and accepts that they have a problem.

Coping with Executive Deficits

1   Recognize the need for increased self-awareness and encourage friends to give you direct feedback about your behaviour. Listen to what others say and identify specific problems to work on.

2   Try to create structure out of unstructured situations. Set yourself goals and then break those goals down into specific tasks so you know what you have to do. Use checklists.

3   Practise training exercises and games which help develop flexible thinking; this includes both divergent thinking (thinking outwards or generating ideas from a single point) and convergent thinking (thinking inwards, taking ideas and summarizing them).

The following exercises not only improve skills but also provide useful feedback, which helps to identify difficulties and improve awareness.

Summarizing the main idea (analysis and convergent thinking)

Read an article from a newspaper, or a paragraph from a book, and then identify the main theme or idea of the article in one sentence. Ask yourself, 'What was that about?' Try not to get side-tracked by details.

Finding information from Yellow Pages (problem solving)

Time yourself on how long it takes you to find the relevant information to solve the following problems: (a) you want to order a cake for a wedding; (b) you want to sell your home; (c) your toilet is blocked; (d) you want to have a picture framed.

Planning projects (planning)

Write down a list of at least seven steps required to achieve the following goals: (a) put a shelf up in the kitchen; (b) change a tyre on a bicycle; (c) move house to a different town; (d) cook a meal for two people.

Expanding categories (divergent thinking)

Name as many items as possible in the following categories in 60 seconds: (a) animals; (b) words beginning with the letter S,F,M,N,P etc; (c) names beginning with M; (d) fruit and vegetables beginning with the letter B,C,T etc; (e) things that have wrinkles; (f) things that hop.

VISUO-SPATIAL AND PERCEPTUAL DIFFICULTIES (MAKING SENSE OF THE WORLD)

Examples of Visuo-spatial and Perceptual Difficulties

1 "I don't seem to be able to judge distances as well as I used to. I might reach out to pick something up and miss it."

2 "I used to be quite good at reading maps; now I am absolutely hopeless."

3 "I don't see things very well on my right-hand side, so I have to turn my head and scan to see them. When reading I have to scan to the end of the line of print, otherwise I'd naturally start reading in the middle of the page."

4 "Sometimes I don't recognize really obvious household items if I see them from a different or unusual angle."

5 "I have great difficulty putting things together. It took me three hours to assemble a roof rack for the car. I also have difficulties with the children's puzzles and jigsaws."

6 "I work in a launderette and I find folding the sheets neatly is now a real problem. I don't know why."

Understanding Perceptual Problems

This group of skills is concerned with understanding and making sense of what we see and hear. The sense organs such as the eyes and ears may be working perfectly well, but the problem occurs when that sensory information is transmitted to the brain. The part of the brain which makes sense of this incoming information is not working properly. These sorts of problems are usually associated with the back half of the brain or the parietal and occipital lobes. The brain's involvement in these skills is sometimes difficult to fully appreciate. Let us take an example. Read the following:

PARIS IN THE

THE SPRING

Did you read the above as 'Paris in the Spring' or did you notice that there were two 'thes' and read it as 'Paris in the the Spring'? The above exercise is a useful way of demonstrating that our impressions or perceptions are largely determined by our brains trying to make sense out of the word rather than our senses such as our eyes. All the examples of problems listed earlier are due, not to faulty eyesight, but to the way the brain organizes the information it receives. There are four main types of perceptual difficulties (see Figure 12):

1   Judging spatial relationships, distance and orientation: this area covers skills such as being able to judge how close a mark is to the middle of a paper, bisecting a line or matching two lines at the same angle.

2   Unilateral neglect: this is often a transitory condition and means that the patient frequently fails to respond to the opposite side of the visual field to where the injury took place. The patient might only read half a line of print, or only shave half his face or, if asked to draw a clock face, might only draw half of it.

3 Object recognition: this is a problem where the person fails to identify and recognize something if it is viewed from a different or unusual angle. This does not just apply to vision but can also affect identification of sounds.

4 Constructional skills: this skill involves putting things together to make something, or building objects from component parts. A particular psychological test called 'block design' is good for teasing this out. The subject is asked to put coloured blocks together to make a particular geometrical design. Very often the person will say, "I know what to do but I just can't do it." Other tasks which require this skill might be to draw a picture of a cube, a star or a bicycle.

Strategies for Improving Perceptual Skills

Perceptual retraining involves recognizing the problem and devising a compensatory strategy or bypassing the damaged area of the brain and using another skill.

1 An important strategy is to encourage scanning — "Look to the left and look to the right." Exercises to improve this skill include (a) counting printed dots scattered on a page of paper, (b) finding a buried object in a complex picture, (c) drawing a coloured line down one side of a page of print and reading across to that line (see box on page 90).

2 Practise copying complex shapes such as a cube, a cross, a star or a word. Try bisecting a line by drawing a line through the middle of two horizontal lines. Practise constructional skills by doing puzzles and jigsaws.

3 Use written visual cues and instructions. If there is a problem dressing, put a list of instructions up on the bedroom wall: 'Touch your left arm'; 'Put your left arm into the shirt'. Eventually the visual and verbal cues can be reduced as the person begins to do it more automatically.

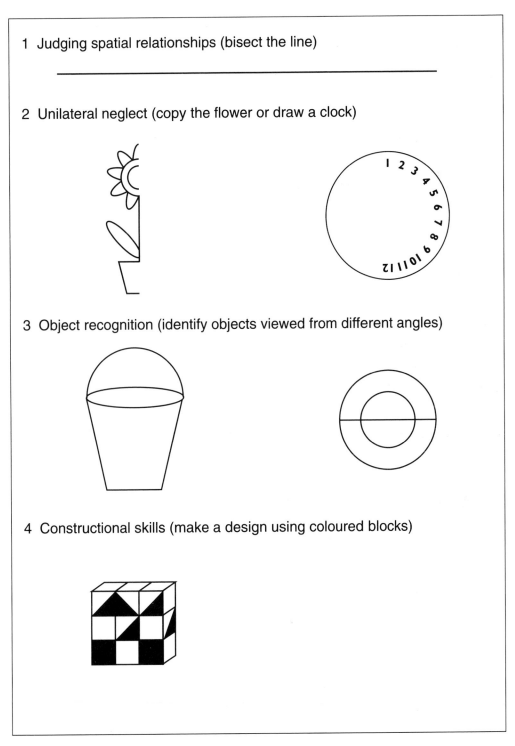

1 Judging spatial relationships (bisect the line)

2 Unilateral neglect (copy the flower or draw a clock)

3 Object recognition (identify objects viewed from different angles)

4 Constructional skills (make a design using coloured blocks)

Figure 12 *Four types of perceptual difficulties*

Why Don't You Finish Your Dinner?
(Understanding Visual Neglect)

"I remember my son saying, 'Mum, why don't you feed me enough?' I said, 'I do, but you always eat half of what's on your plate.' We then began to understand that he was not seeing things in a certain part of his visual field. This meant that when he shaved he only shaved half of his face, when he read a newspaper he could only read the first half of a line, and when he ate he only ate what was on the left-hand side of the plate. It wasn't because his eyesight was poor, it was because the part of his brain that processed that area of information didn't work properly. The difficulty is referred to as a visual neglect or a hemianopia.

"After making that discovery I started marking newspapers with a thick green fluorescent marker-pen down the margin on the right-hand side to make him turn his head and read towards the end of the line. Eventually he became quite good at it and began to turn his head quite naturally to scan." ■

LANGUAGE SKILLS

Examples of Difficulties with Language

1 "Sometimes I just cannot think of the right word. It's on the tip of my tongue but it doesn't come."

2 Marjorie often says the wrong word. For example, yesterday she called a corkscrew a 'bottle screwer', and sellotape 'plaster sticker'.

3 Daniel has great difficulty understanding what people say. We have to speak slowly and use lots of gestures.

4 Alan understands what people say but cannot speak properly. When he does speak his utterances are usually only single words, such as 'No' or 'Yes'. However very rarely, if he gets extremely angry, he can reel off a whole sentence full of swear-words.

5 Karen has great difficulty 'getting to the point' in a conversation — she does not use words precisely or economically.

6 "Peter does not understand me if I talk too quickly or if any sentence has more than three or four sections. If I said, 'Before going to the newsagents, do you think you could go to the greengrocers and buy me some potatoes?' he would not understand. I have to say, 'Go to the greengrocers. Buy some potatoes. Then go to the newsagents', keeping sentences as sequential, short and uncomplicated as possible."

Understanding Language Difficulties

The skills required to hold a conversation are highly complicated. We have to (a) understand what the other person is saying; (b) work out what we want to say; (c) choose the right words with which to respond and put those words in the right order; (d) be able to speak or make sounds; (e) speak at the right volume and speed; and (f) modulate our tone and expression. If certain parts of the brain are injured any one of these stages can become impaired. These types of difficulty with language are often referred to as 'aphasia' or 'dysphasia'. Very simply, there are two main types of 'aphasia': expressive aphasia, which is concerned with talking and expressing ideas in speech, and receptive aphasia, which is concerned with understanding what others are saying. Very often a person may have an expressive aphasia and be unable to speak more than one or two words, but may still be able to understand much of what is said. Alternatively a person may be able to speak but may have difficulties understanding other people, especially if the words used are abstract, or if there is noise or other distractions. When both problems are evident we refer to the condition as being a 'global aphasia'.

One very common problem with expressive aphasia is 'word-finding difficulties'. The person knows the word but cannot find it. He may often say, "The word is on the tip of my tongue." Sometimes he will find a similar word or an approximation of the word that he is looking for. It is like trying to find a book in a library: after some searching you find the right shelf, but then you pick out the wrong book. So instead of calling a picture of a pair of handcuffs by the proper name the person with word-finding difficulty comes up with 'cufflinks', or 'hankers'. This has the effect of restricting the person's vocabulary and often means that his conversation is not as fluent as it might be, or sentences are shorter, words are substituted and circumlocutions occur.

For most people the ability to speak and use language is controlled by the left side of the brain. There is a special area concerned with producing speech (Broca's area, between the frontal and temporal lobe) and another area for understanding the speech of others (Wernicke's area, further back between the temporal and parietal lobes). These two areas are connected by numerous pathways but are quite distinct. Wernicke's area and Broca's area may be separately injured in a stroke, but by the very nature of head injury both are likely to be damaged.

It is useful to remember that these brain skills of producing and understanding speech are different from the ability to produce the actual sounds of language. When people have that problem — their speech is slurred, or too loud, or too quiet — it is often because the muscles in the throat and mouth needed to produce speech are damaged. This is quite usual early on after injury, and with time comes recovery, although some people are left with some permanent difficulty. This difficulty producing the appropriate sounds of speech is known as 'dysarthria' and is often caused by damage to the brain stem, as opposed to 'aphasia', which results from damage to the cerebral cortex.

Exercises for Coping with and Treating Language Difficulties

1. Coping with word-finding difficulties.
   (a) Search your memory in an organized way according to various categories and sub-categories. For example, when trying to think of a person's name, ask yourself, 'Is the person male?'; 'Is the person a member of my family?' Or search letters of the alphabet: 'Does his name begin with A, B, C . . . ?'
   (b) When searching for the name of an object describe it, talk around it, or draw a picture of it. Don't get hung up on getting the word exactly right.
   (c) Create an image of the object in an appropriate scene, then attempt to describe the scene.
   (d) Attempt to generate a sentence using that particular word.
   (e) Use gestures and signs associated with the word.
   (f) Remember that it is getting your message over that matters, not getting the words or sounds exactly right.

2. General advice for helping people with a head injury who have difficulties understanding language:
   (a) Do not speak very quickly; try to use short sentences with familiar words. Accompany your speech with slightly exaggerated gestures and facial expression, and other signs of non-verbal communication. But remember you are talking to an intelligent adult, not a handicapped child.
   (b) Reduce background noise and other distraction.
   (c) Try not to jump from one topic to another in conversation.
   (d) If the person speaks slowly or has difficulty word finding, resist the temptation to speak for them or finish their sentences. Give the person time to put over what they are trying to say.
   (e) Do not pretend that you understand if you do not, as this will lead to frustration for both parties.

(f) If you understand part of what the person is saying, repeat those words back so that they don't have to go through it all again: "You say your mother was born . . . where?"

(g) Watching somebody's lips carefully improves understanding.

3 Examples of tasks used to improve expressive language skills (best carried out under the supervision of a speech therapist):

(a) Describing pictures.

(b) Retelling a short paragraph after somebody else has read it.

(c) Matching words to pictures.

She Can't Speak but She's Not Stupid! (Understanding Expressive Aphasia)

Carol, a 24-year-old girl, had a severe head injury which resulted in an expressive dysphasia, which meant that she was virtually without speech. The only words she could say were 'No' and 'Yes'. She also had a number of other difficulties which meant that she had to live in hospital and have an escort. An inexperienced and rather insensitive nurse escorting Carol to the local Headway centre asked the Headway House co-ordinator a question about Carol, directly in front of her. She said, "What mental age do you think Carol is functioning at?" Carol's response was to stick two fingers up in front of the nurse and storm off. The Headway co-ordinator replied, "Twenty-four years. What's your mental age?"

This true story illustrates three points. Firstly, just because somebody cannot use language does not mean that they do not understand it: the two skills are quite separate and are located in different parts of the brain. Secondly, just because somebody cannot produce speech does not mean that they are necessarily any less intelligent. Thirdly, never speak about a person with a head injury as if they are either stupid or not there. ■

UNDERSTANDING AND COPING WITH EMOTIONAL AND BEHAVIOURAL PROBLEMS

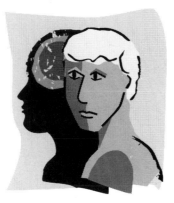

Chapter 6

WHY 'EMOTIONAL AND BEHAVIOURAL PROBLEMS'?

Everybody who has had a head injury is left with some form of emotional and behavioural change. This is inevitable as the brain is the seat and control centre of all our emotions and behaviour. When this complex, delicate piece of equipment is shaken around, emotions and behavioural control will be affected in exactly the same way as thinking, memory, speech and movement are affected. However emotional and behavioural changes are more difficult to see and understand than those other forms of disability. The average man in the street, carer or family member can understand and sympathize with somebody in a wheelchair or on crutches, or even, at a stretch, somebody with speech difficulties or memory problems, but we all find it much harder to understand and accept somebody shouting abuse at us, or acting in a disinhibited or embarrassing way in public. Research suggests that in the long term these emotional and behavioural problems are by far the biggest source of stress to family members.

In the present chapter, I have tried to divide this large, unwieldy topic into a number of different areas, so that, when carers say, "He's just changed and is different", or "His behaviour is a problem", it becomes possible to focus on exactly what the problem is. Once the problem has been broken down and identified, it becomes easier to understand and to identify the best ways of coping. The 12 areas chosen are all interrelated: agitation, explosive anger and irritability, lack of insight and awareness, impulsivity and disinhibition, emotional lability, self-centredness, family abuse, apathy and poor motivation, depression, anxiety, inflexibility and obsessionality, and sexual problems.

Not everybody will have all of these problems; some people may have a few, some people may have many. The severity of these difficulties will also vary; with some people these tendencies will be very obvious, with others they will be less so, and others again will not have the problem at all. Many people go through stages where they may experience these difficulties and then grow out of them.

There seem to be four main reasons as to why these types of difficulty occur: (a) direct neurological damage; (b) exaggeration of previous personality; (c) the stresses of adjustment; and (d) the environment the person lives in.

Direct Neurological Damage

Certain parts of the brain, particularly the frontal lobes, affect the regulation of emotions, motivation, sexual arousal, self-control and self-awareness. Many of the difficulties described in this chapter are characteristics specifically associated with the so-called 'frontal syndrome' or damage to the frontal lobes. Direct damage either by bruising, laceration or shearing means that the delicate balance of neurotransmitters and the highly complex neural pathways, which have developed over the years as we grow to maturity, are disrupted. We all develop from small babies, with little control over our emotions and behaviour, to adults with greater control over these things. Think how a small child acts instinctively and impulsively, crying, screaming and having a temper tantrum whenever the mood dictates. Gradually, just as that child learns to walk, talk, read and write, he learns to control emotions of frustration and anger. Similarly, after a head injury, just as a patient might relearn to walk or talk, he has to relearn emotional control. Sometimes, if the damage is particularly severe, the individual never relearns those old skills and is left with a different temperament or personality.

Exaggeration of Previous Personality

This type of direct neurological damage often has the effect of exaggerating existing personality traits, tendencies and problems that the person had before their injury. It is as if the controls or 'brakes' which modify and regulate the personality have been loosened, and traits and mannerisms become distorted and exaggerated. If the individual was a very restless, outgoing person, they may become more so. If they had a tendency to solve problems by drinking, this may become more pronounced. If they were sexually promiscuous this may become more exaggerated. It is therefore important for professionals to be aware of the patient's previous personality when assessing the factors that are contributing to difficult behaviour.

Stress of Adjustment

Coping with life after a head injury is enormously stressful. Imagine the frustration involved in gradually finding out that you can no longer do the things you used to be able to do. Perhaps the individual forgets simple things, can no longer work as well as before, can no longer play enthusiastically with their children, can no longer compete at their favourite sport, is in pain, constantly feels tired, and is no longer the strong 'breadwinner' in the family, but has rather become dependent on others. It would be bad enough if just one of these things happened, in isolation, but when so many losses and changes occur at the same time the result is enormous frustration, emotional upheaval and stress. When we are under stress it is highly likely that we become more angry and irritable, more anxious and depressed, more preoccupied with our own problems. This stress of adjustment, combined with the effects of direct brain injury, means that these symptoms are exacerbated.

The Environment

The emotional and behavioural reactions of any individual can be influenced by the social and physical environment that a person is in. The social environment includes family, friends, neighbours and professional staff; the physical environment might vary from a ward in a general hospital to a family home. If a person is placed in an environment where their special needs are not understood, communication is poor and there is little love or affection, their behaviour is likely to deteriorate and become inappropriate. All of us become frustrated if somebody does not understand our needs: we may shout louder or sulk, withdraw and become depressed. It is unfortunately true that many people with head injury live in inappropriate environments where their needs are poorly understood. A young 20-year-old girl with a head injury had no supportive family, and so lived on a busy orthopaedic ward in a general hospital for 18 months. Her behaviour became increasingly difficult and she was labelled as a 'behavioural problem'. The majority of the busy nursing staff did not understand her, as they did not have the training, and the physical environment of the hospital was cramped and crowded. When she was eventually transferred to a home in the community her behaviour changed dramatically for the better within a few weeks.

This chapter highlights the 12 key areas of possible emotional and behavioural difficulty in the following way: each section will provide examples of problems, an explanation of why these difficulties might occur and some rough guidelines for coping for carers, and in some cases for the person with the head injury. Some people may recognize and identify with some of these problems, others will not. The guidelines for coping are based on people's experiences and the assumption that some ways of coping can improve a situation, while other ways are likely to make it worse. Whatever the advice, it must be acknowledged that for the carers it is not easy. You need an enormous amount of patience, piles of strength and determination, a rigid backbone to stand firm in the face of increasing demands, and ladles of love and compassion.

AGITATION

Examples

1   "Karen would be constantly getting up and down, moving around, fiddling with things and pacing up and down the ward."

2   "Glynis was restless if left on her own; she would constantly call for the nursing staff, talking continually about going home. She would often start swearing and calling the staff all sorts of names. One day she got so agitated she smashed up her television set."

3   "John continually pulled out his intravenous tube while in hospital."

4 "Mrs Williams became very agitated when relatives or therapists did not arrive at the hospital exactly when expected."

5 "Roy was constantly on the go. He couldn't sit down and be patient, he was up at six o'clock every morning."

Understanding Agitation

Agitation is usually most pronounced in the very early stages after head injury, often while the patient is still in hospital. This type of behaviour is usually unprovoked and unrelated to the person's family or environment. This restlessness and agitation is largely a direct result of neurological damage rather than anything anybody has done. It is important to remember that this is a stage that the patient passes through and not a permanent behaviour change. It is a difficult stage for nursing staff and family members, especially if they do not understand what is happening. Remember that the patient's world has been turned upside down and inside out, leaving them generally confused and disoriented. Often, engaging in agitated behaviour is a way of coping. One patient described this by saying, "I used to walk up and down the corridors. I felt that, if somebody stopped me, I would go crazy."

Coping with Agitation (for Family and Carers)

1 Remember that this is only a stage that the patient is passing through. Be patient.

2 Be available as much as possible during this agitated state, as the patient needs the security of somebody they know.

3 Allow excessive talking — this may be an effective way to work through the agitation.

4 Structure the patient's time so that there are no long periods when they can ruminate.

5 Restructure the environment so that excessive distractions and irritations such as noises are removed and personal effects are installed.

6 Redirect and distract the patient's attention away from the source of agitation. Move the patient gently into new activities. Do not make sudden or quick changes.

7 Model calm behaviour. Appear calm even if you are not.

8 Monitor your own behaviour carefully. Eliminate all verbal and non-verbal cues that could be misinterpreted by the patient (for example, frowning, talking sharply, eye rolling, head shaking, disapproving tone of voice). If you are unaware that you are communicating frustration or anger, ask a friend or colleague to give you feedback.

EXPLOSIVE ANGER AND IRRITABILITY

Examples

1 "I get so annoyed with myself. My temper is on such a short fuse. Sometimes I'll just explode over the silliest things."

2 "I get so irritated with the children and their noise, the television blasting away, or my wife using the vacuum cleaner. I just can't stand the noise and the chaos."

3 "Malcolm is like Jekyll and Hyde. One minute he's all right and then he'll snap over something quite trivial. I'd put his shoes away and he couldn't find them, and it was like a powder keg exploding."

4 "I was a 'bouncer' and doorman in a Glasgow nightclub for eight years, and I prided myself on the fact that I never got into a fight. I'd joke, make people laugh, defuse potentially aggressive situations and would always be in control. Now, since the accident, I wouldn't last a night, as I fly off the handle at the silliest things or if frustrated."

5 "I ended up hitting my own brother with a beer glass and having to take him to hospital. He kept saying stupid things like, 'When are you going back to work, and why can't things be like they used to be?' I told him to leave me alone, but he went on and I just flipped and lost control."

Understanding Explosive Anger and Irritability

Very often in a head injury there is direct damage to the parts of the brain which are involved in controlling emotional behaviour and tolerance of frustration (frontal lobes and limbic system). This often creates emotional lability, meaning that emotions are more likely to swing more extremely and more dramatically. Sometimes this can appear similar to the type of temper tantrums young children have, where an outburst is followed very quickly by calm and even laughter. Just as a child learns to control emotions more effectively, so does the person with the head injury. These difficulties are further exacerbated by the enormous amount of stress and frustration that the head-injured person has to endure as they realize the full extent of their losses. Alongside these difficulties the person with the head injury is less able to filter out distracting, irritating background noise and chaos, which again makes the situation worse.

It is often reported that it is the minor irritations which trigger off the biggest outbursts, such as forgetting a key, an insensitive comment or being kept waiting, rather than major crises. This is because it is the insignificant problems that are the very problems that the individual would have handled so well in the past. The inability to handle these simple tasks uncovers a lack of ability, which is the cause of enormous stress.

Nigel's Story: A Tyrant in His Own Home

Nigel, aged 27, sustained a severe head injury after falling from scaffolding at work. Three years after his accident he still had severe memory and concentration problems, restricted mobility, spending most of his time in a wheelchair, and had developed severe behavioural problems. His elderly parents, with whom he lived, called for professional help. They reported that he was constantly demanding and, if his demands were frustrated, would fly into a terrible temper and threaten to kill himself. Nigel's father, a devout Roman Catholic, when questioned as to why they did not stand up to their son, would say, "What can we do? I'd never forgive myself if he killed himself."

Nigel had become a tyrant in his own house, doing nothing for himself and literally being waited on by caring parents. He liked to play loud pop music, he watched what he wanted on television and had the family video recorder in his room. If his parents tried to stand up to him he would fly into a terrible, frightening rage, with arms and legs going into spasm. His threats of suicide involved wheeling himself into the kitchen to obtain a sharp knife, or wheeling himself to the front door as if to throw himself under traffic. The parents felt they could never leave Nigel alone because, "He's dangerous, his memory is so bad he might leave a cigarette burning, or his mood might go down and he might kill himself."

An outsider can see what has happened in this family and how different factors have interacted, causing a vicious circle to spiral downwards towards the present situation. Nigel's head injury left him demanding, self-centred, very quick to anger and fly into a rage. In the early days after his accident he was very dependent, his parents cared for him, initially doing everything for him, but then they did not stand back and encourage Nigel to do things for himself. Because his parents met all his needs, his tolerance of frustration, which was already low because of the injury, became even lower, to the point where he felt that he could not cope with any frustration. When the parents tried to stand up to Nigel's demands, his rages and threats of suicide played on their guilt feelings and they always gave in. The more he got, the less tolerant he was of frustration, and so the more he demanded. A vicious circle!

The moral for parents and carers is to be firm from an early stage and set boundaries; otherwise you are making a rod for your own back. Nigel could have carried out tasks around the house and certainly could have been left on his own for limited periods of time. Any minimal risk involved would have been well worth it to encourage Nigel's independence. ■

Coping with Anger and Irritability (for Family and Carers)

1   Recognize and, if possible, change the stressors. Spend a week recording on a chart the various situations that trigger or provoke stress and anger. These might include certain discussion topics, people talking too quickly, television or radio being left on, children unexpectedly bringing friends home, or forgetting keys. Now look at ways of reducing the frequency of these stressful events. For example, encourage children in the home to speak more slowly, turn unattended televisions and radios off, avoid certain discussion topics at certain times and have a special hook on the wall by the door for keys.

2   Plan and structure each day and week as much as possible. Life is easier to cope with if it is predictable and regular, rather than being chaotic, with constant unexpected happenings. Try to establish a constant regular rhythm to your lives. Keep a weekly diary or a wall chart. It is easier to cope if you know what is ahead. Negotiate and compromise around the whole family's needs: for example, "The children can have friends around on Tuesday and Friday evenings, but not on other evenings", or "When I vacuum the house, you take the dog for a walk."

Anger Management Training

A Anticipate the trigger situations. Keep a record of when, where and with whom you feel angry or lose your temper. Try to anticipate these triggers by being prepared. Alternatively, alter the situation in some way so that it is less stressful.

N Notice the signs of rising anger. Be aware of those early tell-tale signs of feeling tense and irritable. Notice your muscles tightening up, your breathing speeding up, or your impatience increasing. This is the time to make an alteration in your normal reaction.

G Go through your 'temper routine'. Learn a muscle relaxation exercise; for example, taking a few deep breaths and dropping your shoulders. Repeat to yourself a number of calming statements, such as the three C's: I Calm; stay calm. 2 Challenge; this is a real challenge. 3 Children; they are just children, they can't help it.

E Extract yourself from the situation. If you feel that you are losing the battle to control your temper, leave the situation. Work out, in advance, a number of recognized places to go, or activities; eg. go for a walk, play the piano, or go out into the garden. Physical activity is a good way of burning off the adrenalin which is the fuel of anger.

R Record how you coped. Keep a record of how you coped with each situation. Note which ways of coping were most successful.

3   When appropriate, try gently to redirect and distract the angry person's attention to focus on something more positive.

4   Try not to hold grudges. Make sure there is somebody to talk to about your frustrations.

5   Try not to take it personally. Remember the anger is largely the result of the brain injury. Leave the situation if it gets too much.

LACK OF INSIGHT AND AWARENESS

Examples

1   "Oh yes, everything is fine. We're back to normal, no problems. How are you?"

2   "I haven't got any memory problems; my memory has always been dreadful."

3   "John says that he doesn't want to go on a bus into town because he's tired of buses. But I know that he's very anxious about getting on that bus."

4   "Peter went back to work and tried to carry on as if nothing had happened. He wouldn't admit that he had difficulties until he was given the sack."

5   "George is adamant that he's going to drive again, but he's got poor vision, terrible concentration, a dreadful memory and a foul temper."

6   "When I get better I'm going to do an Open University course."

Understanding Lack of Insight and Awareness

Awareness and insight refer to the ability to be able to understand and judge our own strengths and weaknesses, and to appreciate how our actions are affecting others. This sensitivity to others and the ability to monitor and subtly adjust our own behaviour when appropriate is an important skill which often gets overlooked. Man seems to be the only species in the animal kingdom who possesses this ability to be so self-aware. Not surprisingly these clusters of higher mental skills are thought to be located in the frontal lobes of the brain, and are therefore very likely to be impaired in the majority of closed head injuries. Some people with severe damage to these areas of the brain never fully regain those subtle skills of self-awareness, insight, sensitivity and empathy.

A second reason for the existence of these types of problems is the very nature and circumstances of a traumatic head injury. The majority of people who have had an injury will start off with poor insight and awareness, which will gradually improve over a period of months and years. Just think — we spend our whole lives building up a picture or image of ourselves, we learn about our strengths and weaknesses, we develop expectations, hopes, plans, attitudes and beliefs about ourselves and very suddenly everything is changed. The patient may fully regain consciousness a few days or weeks after the initial injury and find that the physical reality of his world has changed, but his belief and expectations are exactly the same as they have always been. The reality of the situation takes a very long time to sink in and alter the person's beliefs about himself and his future. The situation is perhaps hampered by the fact that the patient may not be able to remember the accident or the traumatic time afterwards. Relatives and carers standing on the touchline, observing broken bodies and experiencing the trauma of their loved one being close to death, have painful memories which in some ways help them to register the full extent of the injury. The person with the injury often misses all that. When consciousness is gradually regained he may be more aware of the most obvious tangible problems, like a stiff shoulder or difficulty moving a leg; then, after a while, he becomes more aware of the subtle cognitive and behavioural problems, and only then does the reality of his disability gradually dawn.

A third factor which contributes to lack of awareness is man's natural tendency to deny the existence of really painful realities as a way of coping and preserving sanity and self-esteem. The process of denial is a natural stage which we all pass through in any loss or bereavement. It is almost as if for our own self-preservation our minds only let us be aware of what we can handle emotionally. In any grieving process denial is naturally replaced by anger, sadness or depression, and finally acceptance.

Coping with Poor Insight (for Family and Carers)

1   Remember that insight and awareness gradually improve and denial is
     a natural way of coping.

2   If the person with the injury wants to engage in an activity that is not
     too dangerous, but you are confident that they will fail, allow them to

do it. Although they may be disappointed, they need to fail to appreciate the reality of the situation and gain insight.

3   When the person with the injury has difficulties and displays problems, draw attention to this in a calm, non-judgemental, non-challenging way. Don't gloat or badger.

4   Try to encourage the patient to join a head injury support group. There will be people at various stages of recovery, and those who have worked through some of their denial may be able to help him recognize and accept his problem areas.

5   Do not be fooled by the person's threats to discontinue occupational therapy or other therapy on the grounds that the tasks are childish. In all likelihood he is experiencing grave difficulty with these tasks, making it all the more important for him to stick with the activity.

6   Involve the individual with the head injury in meetings and decisions about care. Ask professionals to send copies of written reports and assessments to the person with the head injury so he can see exactly what the situation is.

IMPULSIVITY AND DISINHIBITION

Examples

1   "He just grabbed the newspaper out of my hand when I was reading it."

2   "Scott embarrasses me sometimes. He'll say just what he thinks. We were standing in a queue at the supermarket and he started talking, out loud, about how fat and bald the man in front of us was."

3 "Martin will touch people inappropriately — putting his arm around total strangers as if they were lifelong friends."

4 "I know Freud said we are all supposed to think about sex all the time, but Alan talks about it all the time. He'll say the crudest things."

5 "If Roy disappears I look for the nearest person standing still and he'll be talking to them. They think he's off his head. That's what hurts."

6 "He stood in the middle of Tesco's shouting at me at the top of his voice."

7 "Michael is like a 25-year-old child. If he goes into a shop and he wants some sweets he'll just help himself and often walks out without paying. He doesn't think through the consequences of his actions."

Understanding Impulsivity and Disinhibition

Impulsivity and disinhibition are the lack of ability to control either actions or speech. The person will act on impulse, will say the first thing that comes into his head and will express feelings, thoughts and opinions without weighing up the consequences. It is as if the normal 'brake' or 'censor' that controls our behaviour is not working. The person responds to anything and everything equally, and does not seem to be able to judge carefully, weigh up options or filter out inappropriate actions. These difficulties are due to neurological damage in the areas of the frontal lobes.

These characteristics are not only frustrating but also very embarrassing for the family. Impulsivity leads to excessive 'demanding behaviour', which can be both tiring and irritating. The problem is made worse because this behaviour usually goes hand in hand with lack of awareness, so the person with the head injury blurts out the first thought that enters his head, regardless of who is present. While the family is mortified the person does not appear to comprehend the significance of the breach of etiquette.

Coping with Impulsivity and Disinhibition (for Family and Carers)

1   Recognize that the person's problem is due to the brain injury. Try to understand it.

2   Give the person firm, direct verbal feedback when he behaves inappropriately: "No, Martin. It is inappropriate for you to kiss my hand."

3   Devise a behavioural management system. Ask for help from professionals, such as a psychologist. The system involves making sure that all actions have either a positive or a negative consequence. Periods of appropriate behaviour are followed by rewards, and negative behaviour is followed by withdrawal of rewards. Rewards might be ticks on a chart, tokens, which can be exchanged for presents, money, or praise and attention.

4   Redirect the patient's attention to appropriate behaviour. For example, Frank would often question people about intimate aspects of their sex life. This was met with a comment stressing the inappropriate nature of the conversation and then distracting him with another topic of conversation.

5   Be quite strict early on. Don't allow impulsive behaviour to be rewarded or reinforced. This means trying to prevent a pleasant consequence occurring after the impulsive action. Do not make exceptions and say, "Oh that's just Martin. He likes to touch people." Be firm, set boundaries and limitations and spell out the fact that the behaviour is inappropriate. The consequence of not being firm is that the person's lack of control over his behaviour increases. The individual may start off touching and then progress to kissing and may then find he has developed a habit which becomes very difficult to break.

EMOTIONAL LABILITY

Examples

1 "Peter only has to start talking about our grandchildren and he starts to cry."

2 "Ralph will cry openly when discussing how kind and thoughtful the nursing staff have been. Two minutes later he will be laughing again."

3 "Jeff will laugh and giggle before every comment he makes, regardless of how funny it is."

4 "Tony just does not seem to feel things deeply any more — his emotions are shallow — he has no empathy."

Understanding Emotional Lability

Emotional lability means nothing more than loss of control over emotions. The fact that the emotions are more quickly displayed does not necessarily mean that the emotion is stronger than it was. Instead the person has lost the ability to discriminate about when and how to express his feelings. While most people can control their expression of joy, sadness or anger, and limit it to the right time and place, the person with the brain injury cannot. This difficulty is directly due to damage to the brain, especially the areas dealing with impulses and emotions. These quick and frequent mood swings can be extremely tiring for family members who are trying to keep things on an even keel. As time progresses it is usual for the person with the head injury to relearn increasing emotional control.

Coping with Emotional Lability (for Family and Carers)

1 Do not criticize the person with a head injury, as their increased sensitivity is likely to lead to an excessive over-reaction.

2   Point out and praise occasions when they do manage to control their emotions. At those times identify and discuss how they managed to maintain self-control. Encourage them to use those strategies again.

3   Try to model calm behaviour yourself.

4   Realize that the person with the head injury will have difficulty coping with even mild stress. Attempt to structure the environment so that unnecessary stress factors are removed.

SELF-CENTREDNESS

Examples

1   "Peter wanted to watch a particular TV programme and, even though nobody else in the family wanted it, he demanded that we watch it."

2   "He never says to me, 'Did you have a nice day?' He's so wrapped up in his own problems he's not interested in anybody else."

3   "He will just sit in the same room as my son, but will not think to play with him or even talk to him. It's a pity because they used to be so close and previously he would be down on the floor playing with the kids."

4   "I look after him all day and occasionally I need to get out of the house. I try to pop out to the social club, maybe one evening a week. He resents it and tries to stop me, saying, 'You don't really care.' If he cared about me he'd encourage me to go out."

5   "He doesn't take an interest in the news, or what's happening in the family, whereas before he'd always read the newspapers and discuss current events."

Understanding Self-centredness

After a severe head injury, the patient often becomes completely self-centred, displaying behaviour similar to that of a three- or four-year-old. The world revolves around them. This is partly due to direct brain injury, restricting the patient's ability to be aware and insightful of his own and others' behaviour, and the ability to be able to put himself in somebody else's shoes. The specific ability to empathize, or imagine how somebody else is feeling, is a high-level sophisticated mental skill. Again these skills are located in the frontal lobes, the area which is often damaged. Alongside these deficits the patient may actually have difficulty picking up subtle social cues, as in recognizing when a child wants to talk or play with his daddy. Apart from the problems caused by direct neural damage it must be remembered that the patient has had a terrible experience which is enormously stressful and will be all-consuming and preoccupying. He will also need to talk about it to release the tension.

Inadvertently families can often encourage self-centredness. Following the trauma the family is so overjoyed that their loved one is alive that it is easy to spoil him. Initially everything is geared to the needs of the person with a head injury. This is when family members need to be strong and recognize that their own needs are as important: to say, "Yes, I'll get you that when I've finished what I'm doing", rather than jumping up immediately and responding to all demands.

Unfortunately, if this trait of self-centredness is too severe, it is often the 'crowning blow' to efforts by family members to reintegrate the person into the home environment. We are all very willing to go the extra mile for someone who realizes and appreciates our efforts, but are less inclined to be responsive to selfish individuals. As a result, families and friends often pull away, which in turn often results in the person becoming more egocentric. It is unfortunately true that friends and social networks tend to disintegrate six months after the injury. This is another behavioural problem that does not cure itself, and in fact can worsen if appropriate steps are not taken.

Coping with Self-centredness (for Family and Carers)

1   Do not relinquish everything to meet the needs of the person with the injury.

2   Do not allow the person to get to the point where they expect that all their demands will be met.

3   Avoid the trap of doing everything for him, or always being there. This can often encourage the person with a head injury to be disabled. Allow them to do things even if it takes longer.

4   Do not expect the person to respect your rights. You may have to do some demanding of your own. You have to look after your own needs — be assertive.

5   Encourage him to get involved with a head injury support group. Often the best way to get somebody to realize his own fault is to see it in someone else and thus criticize selfishness.

FAMILY ABUSE

Examples

1   "Jamie is so sweet and nice to the nurses, yet at home he's a devil. He's rude, critical, irritable, mentally and physically abusive. It's almost as if he saves up all his bad behaviour for us."

2   "Peter threatened his mother with a knife when she refused to let him use her car."

3   "He sits at home staring at me and accuses me of having an affair. It's like being tortured."

4   "He's so intolerant of me. I can't do anything right."

5   "Tony knocked his dinner off the table and shouted at his mother, 'What's this slop?'"

6   "Dad won't let me bring Mark, my fiance, into the house now. They never got on before his accident, but now he hates him."

Understanding Family Abuse

This is the age-old story of 'You only hurt the ones you love', in that family members often receive the major portion of the abuse the person with the head injury has to offer. At first, immediately after the injury, the patient will have little control over his behaviour and may be abusive to anyone and everyone. As he begins to develop some behavioural control, he becomes more socialized with staff, friends and strangers. With effort, he can control his impulses in these social situations. However, at home or with family, where he has always been more relaxed, never having to make an effort or put on a show, he continues to behave in an abusive manner. It is not that he is any meaner than before the injury, but he is just responding more spontaneously.

Also those closest to the person with a head injury are 'safe targets', in the sense that, because they love the person, they will take the abuse without withdrawing or turning away. Sometimes the person with a head injury needs that safety-valve to vent his frustration and rage.

Family abuse can often create real difficulties at home. Families often find themselves compromising and avoiding anything that may 'set him off'. They change many things to please him. As the person with the head injury becomes more aware of his actions, there is always the danger that he may manipulate and control family members. This transition is often gradual, so that no one realizes that the situation has changed from the person with the head injury being completely out of control to the individual controlling everyone's behaviour.

Coping with Family Abuse (for Family and Carers)

1 Don't take it personally. Remember you are a 'safety-valve' or 'safe target' which the head-injured person needs.

2 Try to treat each occurrence as an isolated incident. He might not remember or be aware that he acted in this way before.

3 Do not allow yourself to live under a 'reign of terror'. Succumbing to the person's threats may set up a pattern that could take years to break.

4 Remember that most threats are expressions of anger, frustration and fear of a situation rather than at an individual.

5 If young children are involved, help them to recognize and avoid behaviour that could be potentially harmful. If there is a high risk that young children may be harmed, it may be best to remove them from the situation.

6 Maintain some type of outside support (counsellor or friend) to express your feelings.

7 Educate all family members to respond to abusive threats consistently. If the person with the head injury learns that he can get the desired response from one person and not another he will quickly learn to manipulate the person who has given in.

Apathy and Poor Motivation

Examples

1 "Jeff just sits in front of the television all day. He doesn't do anything. He's got no enthusiasm. Before he was always on the go, planning holidays and racing around."

2 "Richard used to be very interested in stamp collecting but he now shows no spark of interest."

3 "We used to go out at least five nights a week. Now Sam just sits in and does jigsaws."

4 "Since I had my head injury I sometimes think, 'I want to do a thousand different things, but I don't get around to doing any'."

5 "He's not as sharp and tenacious as he used to be. He's lost his drive."

Understanding Apathy and Poor Motivation

Lack of motivation or spontaneity, or apathy is a direct result of brain injury to frontal lobe structures that concern emotion, motivation and forward planning. The person with the head injury may be motivated to have immediate needs gratified, saying such things as "I want food", "I want quiet", "I want to be comfortable", but sustained, planned motivation is more difficult. Often the person is unable to conceptualize and plan activities, or work towards specific goals, because cognitive abilities involving planning are injured. Often these goals are so overwhelming that it is less threatening and less anxiety-provoking to just sit and ruminate. Working towards a goal requires planning, realistic appraisal of the situation and self-appraisal, and these are the very skills that are often impaired. As time passes, this lack of motivation can lead to relative social isolation, lack of pleasure and, at times, depression. This lack of initiative and spontaneity is often very frustrating for families and carers. Beware of confusing apathy and poor motivation with tiredness and fatigue.

Coping with Apathy and Poor Motivation (for Family and Carers)

1   At times be firm and say to the person with a head injury, "We are going to . . .", rather than asking, "Do you want to . . . ?", or give him a choice between two desirable activities.

2   Break down the activities into small steps to avoid overwhelming the individual: "Get your clothes on"; then, "Have breakfast"; then, "Come with me to the supermarket."

3   Work out a behavioural management system. This simply means changing the payoffs for certain activities. Reward and reinforce certain desired activities and withdraw rewards for undesirable other activities.

4   Encourage involvement in a support group. This leads to stimulation and encouragement from others with similar difficulties.

DEPRESSION

Examples

1   "I feel so down. What's the point? I can't work properly. I can't stand being with my kids. I'm always upsetting my wife."

2   "I should have died in the accident, it would have been better for everybody."

3 "Terry sleeps until midday, then just sits in front of the TV. He's angry at everybody, but will not talk about it."

4 "The only time I can forget about how bad things really are is when I've had a drink."

5 "I've always been such a hard-driving person, always working towards achieving something, such as passing exams, and earning more money. Now there is a big void. I know I'll never work again and I feel absolutely useless."

Understanding Depression

Depression is a very common emotional reaction which comes later on in the stages of rehabilitation. Depression usually surfaces when the person with the head injury begins to realize the full extent of his losses. This often occurs after formal rehabilitation is over, when the person has gone home. There is a realization that life can never be like it was before. It might be that the activities that previously produced pleasure are no longer possible. This might include high standards at work, sporting activities, mobility, being quick-witted, being sexually attractive, writing, reading or being the breadwinner. But often depression is a good sign because it is actually a sign of progress. The person has become progressively more aware of the reality of his situation and is digesting the emotional consequences. To reach a level of real adjustment and acceptance it may well be necessary to work through this painful trough of depression. It is useful to distinguish between the normal, healthy type of depression, where the individual is overwhelmingly sad, pessimistic and is actively grieving for the many losses he has to adjust to, and a depressed state where the person is emotionally blocked and is unable to express his feelings openly. The latter state may benefit from professional counselling from somebody who knows about head injury.

Coping with Depression (for the Carer)

1   If suicidal thoughts are expressed take them seriously and seek professional help.

2   Adopt diversionary tactics to get his mind off depressive thoughts.

3   Do not take responsibility for the depression — it is not your fault.

4   Do not remind the person with the head injury of his progress by reiterating how bad he used to be. This will only make him feel worse.

Coping with Depression (for the Person with the Head Injury)

I   Talk it through with somebody who is a good listener.

2   Express your feelings. Do not bottle them up.

3   Get involved in a head injury support group and talk to others in a similar situation. Find out how they cope.

4   Involve yourself in any activity that brings pleasure. Try to stay active. Break large tasks down into smaller tasks.

5   Lower your expectations. Work towards enjoying the pleasure of the moment rather than the pleasure of achievements.

ANXIETY

Examples

1   "Marjorie gets so anxious and panicky if she's in a new or unusual situation."

2   "He won't go anywhere without me."

3   "I was in a crowded pub with my girlfriend and some of her friends. I came over all funny, feeling very dizzy, my heart started beating really quickly, and I just had to get out. I suppose it was a panic attack."

4   "He keeps asking, 'Where have you been?' and 'When will you be back?' He hates being left on his own for even the briefest amount of time."

5   "Claire becomes almost rigid with fear when she has to be a passenger in somebody else's car."

6   "I just feel really nervous about so many things, from answering the phone to walking down the street. I also wake up with terrible night-mares."

Understanding Anxiety

It is natural for people who have been involved in a traumatic experience to feel anxious afterwards. If a person has been assaulted, or involved in a road traffic accident, going back into the original situation is likely to increase anxiety. However that anxiety will die away with time. Longstanding problems and phobias can occur if the person continues to avoid those situations rather than face his fears.

General symptoms of stress and anxiety, such as panic attacks, worry and tension, are also common. Undoubtedly, life after a head injury is enormously stressful. Imagine being inactive for a lengthy period when medically ill, then attempting to get 'back to normal' and finding that there are so many things that you cannot do as well as you could before the injury. Confidence is at a low level, and the world becomes a frightening, distressing place. Adjustment to this new situation takes time. Feelings of anxiety and depression are normal.

In the early stages after a severe injury, the patient is naturally dependent on family and professional carers. However, over time, the person changes, learning to do more things for himself. It is important at this point for carers to 'step back' and encourage independence, even though the individual at times may be inclined to 'cling on' to the safety and security of the carer. There is a fine line between being helpful and encouraging independence, and doing too much for the person and allowing him to become dependent. If he becomes dependent, his anxiety about going into new situations will stay high, and his confidence in his own ability will remain low.

Coping with Anxiety (for the Person with the Head Injury)

1   Talk about your fears, worries and anxieties. Ventilate your feelings. Do not bottle them up. Talk to other people in similar situations; join a head injury support group.

2   Learn ways of relaxing and staying calm. This might include learning an anxiety management technique such as muscle relaxation, slow breathing, distracting yourself from worrying thoughts, positive thinking or yoga.   If the problem is too great, seek professional advice from a clinical psychologist or counsellor with knowledge of head injury.

3   Try not to avoid difficult situations that make you feel anxious. The more you push yourself and face the fear, the quicker the anxiety will disappear.

4   Do not be too hard on yourself. Things have changed in your life. Perhaps you can no longer do some of the things that you used to do, but unfortunately your expectations are telling you that you still can. Those high expectations need lowering; this is emotionally painful and will create anxiety.

Coping with Anxiety (for Family and Carers)

1   Do not let yourself become the only friend of the person with the head injury.

2   Try not to do things for him. Encourage as much self-sufficiency as possible. Encourage him to go out on his own.

3 Encourage him to meet new people, one at a time. Do not push him into a large group which is completely overwhelming.

4 Set simple tasks to begin with, and then, when he feels confident, make them progressively more difficult. Confidence is built by small successes. For example, a first step might be: "Go into a shop and buy a newspaper"; gradually work up to the most difficult situation, which might be: "Catch a bus into town, on your own and buy some clothes."

INFLEXIBILITY, RIGIDITY AND OBSESSIONALITY

Examples

1 "John's mind is so set firm, it's like concrete. It is no use talking to him."

2 "He is so unreasonable, so black and white. He won't accept that he's wrong. Before, he was always more relaxed and could see both sides of an argument."

3 "Mike is obsessed with problems he can't solve. He keeps going on about his business and the people that owe him money. But, realistically, that's all in the past now — he doesn't even have a business."

4 "Dawn hoards toys, possessions, games, and won't go out without carrying certain things."

5 "Every day for the last two years Dave asks me when I think he'll be better and able to go to work."

6 "Jack has to try to do all the decorating himself although he is really not capable. He stubbornly refuses to pay for somebody else to do it. Then, when he is doing it, it takes him ages and makes him incredibly frustrated because he can't do it to his high standards."

7 "She is constantly washing her hands and checking things."

Understanding Inflexibility and Obsessionality

This type of rigid behaviour is rather like tunnel vision, when the person with the head injury becomes obsessed by a particular idea or thought and grinds it into the ground. The roots of this problem are again cognitive difficulties caused by direct neurological injury to the frontal lobes. The individual has difficulty 'switching' from one line of thought to another. Thinking becomes more rigid, or 'concrete'. The person loses the power to jump from one idea to another and often becomes 'stuck' on one particular thought. If the person has memory problems the situation can be exacerbated as he may forget what he has already said or done. It is also worth bearing in mind that these obsessional patterns of behaviour are more likely to surface if the person is feeling particularly anxious or insecure. This type of behaviour can be particularly irritating to family and friends, and is often one of the factors that lead to social isolation.

Coping with Inflexibility and Obsessionality (for Family and Carers)

1 Try to understand the behaviour and, if possible, ignore it.

2 Redirect attention to new ideas and more constructive behaviour.

3 Reassure the person. This type of behaviour is often the result of anxiety, so alleviating the underlying fear will help him move on to other thoughts.

4   Do not confront or belittle the behaviour; this will often only lead to more anxiety and further obsessions.

SEXUAL PROBLEMS

Examples

1   "Since my accident I'm just not interested in sex any more. I just don't feel anything."

2   "Since his accident Gavin wants to make love every night. It's a real problem because I don't want to."

3   "John misinterprets people's actions. He was insistent that one of the staff fancied him because, in his words, 'She wiggled her tongue at me.' But I would bet any money that she was just licking her lips."

4   "Martin is always touching people and making sexual innuendo and off-colour remarks. He really embarrasses people."

5   "Jerry desperately wants a girlfriend. The trouble is that he is just too impatient and impulsive. He only has to have one conversation, or even just a smile, and he's asking them to marry him."

6   "Since her accident Angela has become quite promiscuous, and people do take advantage of her."

Understanding Sexual Problems

The sexuality of the person who has experienced a head injury can be either increased or decreased, as the result of physical damage or for a variety of psychological reasons. There is a small nerve centre in the middle of the brain, called the hypothalamus, which regulates sex drive and the release of testosterone. If this is damaged, sexual appetite may either increase or decrease. Psychological factors creating sexual difficulties include the person feeling unattractive, feeling continuously tired, or having a strong fear of rejection. In other cases roles within the family may have changed significantly; the dominant, male 'breadwinner', may now be in the completely different role of dependant and need 'looking after'. The person with the head injury, and/or his partner, may feel this role is incompatible with sexual activity.

A second problem area is often inappropriate sexual behaviour. If the person with the head injury is slightly disinhibited, has little awareness of the effects of his own behaviour, is a young male with a normal sex drive and, because of the complications of his injury, does not have a girlfriend, then there invariably will be difficulties. These problems are often exacerbated by the patient misinterpreting the sexual behaviour of others, or being very impatient, impulsive and 'black-and-white' in their thinking. One young man, who had a severe head injury, but had made a good recovery over five years and had a part-time job in a supermarket, noticed that one of the check-out girls was very friendly towards him. He interpreted this as a 'come on' and approached her with a packet of condoms, saying, "I've got a packet of three here and know how to use them." The girl was very upset, complained to her manager and the young man lost his job. The problem was due partly to his misinterpretation of 'social cues', partly to his disinhibition and partly to rigid 'black-and-white' thinking. The subtleties and niceties of courting rituals, where a couple goes through various stages of getting to know each other, often get jettisoned by the impatient, impulsive rigid-thinking patient, who wants to move straight to 'level five' and miss out all the early stages.

Coping with Decreased Sexual Interest (for the Partner)

1   Do not take your partner's lack of interest personally.

2   Do not pressurize or embarrass your partner into a sexual relationship prematurely.

3   Remember that the lack of interest may be a 'smoke screen' for a lack of confidence in ability to perform.

4   Talk openly about the problem and share it with each other. Jointly try experimenting with magazines or videos of an erotic nature — see whether there is any arousal.

Coping with Increased or Inappropriate Sexual Interest (for the Partner)

1   The person should be told as often as necessary and as clearly as possible that certain inappropriate behaviour is not acceptable.

2   If the person does not curtail the behaviour, it should be treated like any other inappropriate or aggressive behaviour, with loss of privilege, isolation and restraint.

3   Encourage the individual to become involved in a support group where he will become more aware of the consequences of this behaviour and can regain confidence in his social abilities.

4   If your partner's sexual appetite has increased to inappropriate levels, do not feel obliged to respond to sexual demands every time. You have the right to say when and how often you want to engage in sexual activity.

5 Whatever the nature of the sexual problem, it often helps to speak to a counsellor, psychologist or social worker who has some understanding of head injury.

Social Skills Training

Loss of good social skills is a crucial problem for people with head injury and their families. Social skills are being able to get on with other people, expressing oneself openly and relating in a smooth, appropriate manner. Inadequate skills lead to poor relationships, difficulties at work, loss of friendships, loneliness, embarrassment and stress for others. We can all improve our social skills to some extent. We know that brain injury, especially to the frontal lobe areas, causes impulsivity, disinhibition, lack of insight, poor judgement and difficulty in self-monitoring; it is these difficulties which in turn produce social skills problems.

Types of Social Skills Problems

1   Francis stands much too close to people when he speaks.
2   Martin constantly interrupts other people's conversation when they are talking.
3   Jane talks too loudly, in a monotonous tone.
4   Brian talks excessively without allowing the listener to get a word in edgeways and he never picks up the cue that they may want to speak.
5   Mary has lost her confidence in talking in front of a group.

Training

A social skill, like any other skill, can be learned. To learn a skill a person needs to recognize, identify and describe the skill that they lack and want to acquire. One technique is as follows:

1   An instructor demonstrates the skill and acts as a model.
2   The trainee then practises and rehearses the skill.
3   The instructor gives feedback and shapes the trainee's performance.
4   The trainee then deliberately practises that skill in the outside world.

Social skills training can be carried out individually or in groups. Modelling, role-playing and giving constructive feedback are important components of the approach. Video feedback has also been shown to be effective.

HEAD INJURY:
A FAMILY AFFAIR

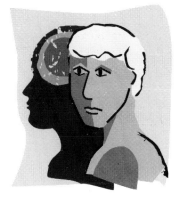

Chapter 7

STRESSES ON THE FAMILY

It is frequently said that there are not just head-injured individuals but rather head-injured families, because the whole family is affected. Some would say that families are the real victims and often suffer more than the head-injured person because they are more likely to have accurate insight into the problem. No family is ever prepared and ready for a head injury; most families already have a full agenda of problems to cope with before clearing the decks to cope with the problems of head injury. Research into the effects of severe head injury on the other family members gives some indication of the extent of their difficulties. The following points are worth noting:

1 Close family members are likely to experience high levels of anxiety and depression during the years following a head injury. As time elapses, there is often a decrease in relatives' capacity for coping, particularly with emotional and behavioural problems.

2 Spouses often feel isolated and trapped with a marriage where their emotional needs are not being met. Some describe this as being neither married nor single. Relationships are put under enormous strain, and it is estimated that between 20 and 50 per cent of all marriages in which one spouse has had a severe head injury end in divorce.

3 Children often experience emotional problems as, alongside coping with the initial trauma, and the subsequent difficult behaviour of a parent with a head injury, their own needs are often neglected, and this can impair their performance at school.

Families need attention, education, guidance and support if they are to survive, regroup and rebuild their lives. Some families cope better than others, but all have difficulties. There is no normal way of responding to a head injury. The saying that 'people act abnormally in abnormal situations' is undoubtedly appropriate.

The people in families and relationships who seem to cope best are those that have two special qualities: first, the ability to be flexible, not being rigidly tied to how things ought to be, but being able to embrace change and view it as a challenge; and second, the ability to communicate openly and honestly, directly expressing emotions both positive and negative, and recognizing the needs of themselves and others within the family. If a family has these characteristics of flexibility and open communication, then it is possible that, out of the crisis of head injury, a family can grow in strength through its way of dealing with it. The fragility of life can give a whole new perspective and intensity to the love that existed prior to the head injury. Having a person with disability in the family often brings a new sensitivity and awareness to other members of the family. It is often said that the experience of head injury tends to make strong marriages and relationships stronger, and troubled relationships more troubled.

THE FAMILY'S STAGES OF EMOTIONAL REACTION

The family close to the person who has had a severe head injury embarks on an emotional roller-coaster, where emotions rise and fall as expectations soar and plummet. Coping with a head-injured relative is not as straightforward as coping either with illnesses where there is a cure or with death, where there is a final resolution. In death the enormous loss is final and very obvious. The loved one has gone and relatives then have time to grieve and mourn. Rituals such as funerals help that grieving process. Family members go through a well recognized range of emotions, from shock, denial and anger to sadness and acceptance. However, with head injury, because of the long-drawn-out process of recovery and rehabilitation the emotions associated with loss come and go in recurring cycles. One day a relative may feel grief at all the losses, and the next day expectations may dramatically rise because the person has made a step forward, and the emotion of grief is temporarily shelved.

It often takes a very long time for individuals to accept that their loved one is not going to 'get back to normal'. The familiar body is there, but there are many changes, most of which are losses. At the same time as the members of the family are trying desperately to cope with feelings of loss, they also have to react to the everyday events and difficulties associated with head injury. These include coping with the cognitive, behavioural and social problems, lack of information and services, uncertainty about the future, possible financial difficulties and role changes. Just as the person with the head injury goes through various stages of recovery and acceptance, so does the family (see Figure 13). It is helpful to map out the different stages of emotional reaction families are likely to go through.

Stage one lasts from the time of injury to medical stabilization. The family's initial emotional reaction is usually a mixture of shock, panic, disbelief and denial. Their main concern is with the survival of their loved one: "Please God, let him live."

Stage two occurs when the patient regains consciousness. At this time the family experiences relief, elation and often massive denial about future realities. There is a tendency to focus on minor improvements in order to justify often unrealistic beliefs about recovery. In these early days the family often do not want to know anything about Headway, head injury, or head injury support groups.

Stage three typically coincides with the period of rehabilitation, and family members may maintain a hopeful attitude. However during the latter part of this stage they may begin to become discouraged and concerned by slow progress. At this point the family member may experience a mixture of anxiety, anger, guilt and depression, which may be expressed in anger towards professionals.

Stage four is often precipitated by a return to the community and discharge from rehabilitation services. Awareness of the probable permanence of impairments and the realization that there will be little further change produce feelings of depression, anger and grief.

Stage five can be said to be the relative's emotional acceptance and realistic recognition of the person with the injury's limitations. This is perhaps a point on the horizon that people work towards and never quite reach — a long journey, rather than a destination.

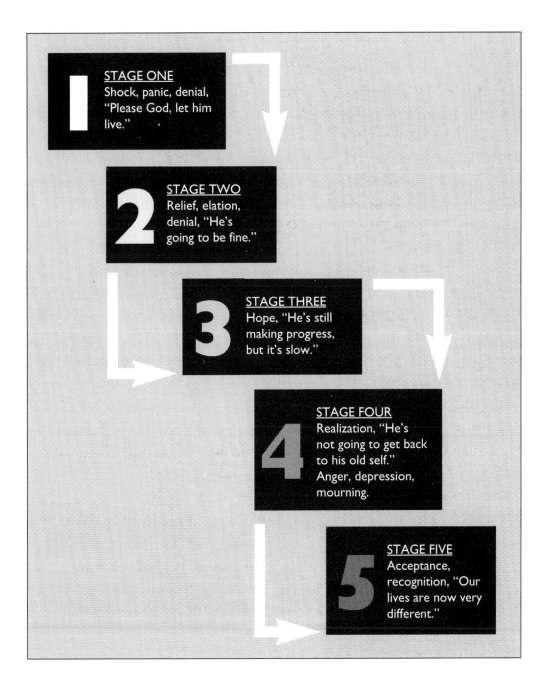

Figure 13 *The stages of the family's emotional reaction*

WAYS OF HELPING THE FAMILY (FOR PROFESSIONALS AND HELPERS)

Relatives will have contact with a range of professionals and, it is hoped, members of a head injury support group. Obviously some will know more about head injury than others. It is important to bear in mind that professionals who work in one particular specialist field may not have a full understanding of the broad and long-term effects of head injury. Other families and relatives who have been through the various stages of emotional reaction, from initial shock to long-term adjustment, can be especially helpful and supportive. A number of guidelines and roles for helpers are worth considering.

1 Professional hospital staff should be very sensitive about their initial encounter with families because this tends to set the tone for future encounters. Giving negative information which is not borne out by subsequent developments may lead the family to develop disbelief in all information given by professionals. After all, if they have proved the professionals wrong once, why not again? Professionals need to be open and honest, acknowledging that it is a difficult time to talk to families, avoid being too negative, refrain from making predictions about the future, especially negative ones and be willing to say "I don't know", if they are in any doubt.

2 Provide information and education to the family such as booklets and pamphlets about the effects of head injury, and the range of services available. The family is often confused and overwhelmed. However, bear in mind the different stages that the head-injured person and his family may have reached. Tailor the information to the right stage. Help the family to gradually adjust their expectations.

3 Help the family members to express and communicate their feelings of anger, guilt, frustration and grief. Normalize these feelings: "It is normal to

react in this way."

4 Help identify the different role changes that need to occur in the family. For example, the person with the head injury may not be capable of full-time employment, or may not be able to deal with bills and family finance. Provide practical management advice. Encourage the family members to recognize the importance of considering the needs of the whole family, particularly those of younger children.

5 Advocacy and advice. The family may need practical help and advice concerning such areas as claiming allowances, litigation and compensation, rehabilitation centres, work assessments, assessing local statutory services, joining local self-help groups and so on.

The rest of the chapter looks at a number of difficult emotions and situations that the family are likely to experience. It must be pointed out that everybody responds differently and not everybody will experience all the following emotions or difficulties. However, as in the previous chapter, these potential difficulties are worth pointing out; the intention is to give a few examples of the experience, then attempt to understand the phenomenon, and finally to offer a few broad suggestions for coping.

Anxiety and Panic

Examples

1 The wife of a man with an injury gets irate and shouts when a doctor has not shown up on time.

2 A mother refuses to visit her son in hospital for the first two weeks, being frozen with panic, then on her first visit starts shaking uncontrollably and crying.

3   Parents spend every waking moment frantically stimulating their son, who is in a coma.

4   Parents panic if anticipated goals are not reached. The doctor may have said, "If he wakes up in two weeks his chances of recovery will be better", but there is still no sign of consciousness.

5   A wife gets very anxious over a planned holiday, constantly asking, "Will he be better in time?"

Understanding Anxiety and Panic

The first reaction is often panic, followed by disorientation, inability to concentrate and an extreme feeling of loss of control. This usually occurs until the patient is declared medically stable. Often relatives say to themselves, "If only he lives, that's all that matters." However the closer the patient gets to safety, the greater are the family's requirements. Once it is evident that the patient will live, relatives focus on his progressing ability to eat, to walk, to talk, to care for himself, and finally to return to work. Anxiety levels constantly fluctuate around the achievement of these different stages.

Coping with Anxiety and Panic

1   Ask questions about what is going on in the hospital. What is that machine doing? Asking for explanations is important, as knowing something about what is happening helps the family feel involved and less anxious.

2   Acknowledge the fact that, in the early medical stages, the situation is out of your hands. Do not try to take control; this will only lead to more frustration and panic.

3   Redirect your energies to those areas where you can have an impact, such as support of other family members, or care of dependent children.

4   Do not set arbitrary goals or expectations during the stage of medical stabilization.

5   Keep communicating and expressing yourself. Don't bottle it up.

6   Learn some relaxation techniques from a counsellor or psychologist. Alternatively buy a book or tape about relaxation.

7   Deliberately take time for yourself. Give yourself permission to take part in a relaxing or pleasurable activity.

8   Don't try to be everything to everybody. Delegate responsibility to others. People often want to help but do not know how.

9   Prioritize — there are some things that just are not that important.

10   Stay clear of people who provoke anxiety.

Denial and Over-optimism

Examples

1   The family tells the patient that they will buy him a new car for his birthday.

2   The family says to the patient, "Don't worry, son, you'll be back to work by Christmas."

3   The wife excuses her husband (the patient) by saying, "He's always had a bad memory" or "He's always had a short temper."

4   A wife discourages her husband from going for further rehabilitation, or going to the Headway day centre, because "He's not really as bad as a lot of those people."

Understanding Denial and Over-optimism

Denial is a natural defence mechanism which helps us to cope with intense, painful emotions. It allows bad news to seep in a little at a time. Similarly there is nothing wrong with optimism for keeping the spirits up, but there does come a point where denial and over-optimism can adversely affect the patient's rehabilitation and progress. Denial by family members, combined with lack of insight in the patient, can produce an unwillingness to face up to the negative affects of the trauma. If problems are not recognized they cannot be helped or overcome. A symptom of denial is 'doctor shopping', or deciding that the opinions of the rehabilitation team are inaccurate, and looking for a different opinion.

Coping with Denial and Over-optimism

1   Take it one day at a time. Deal with today's problems without letting your expectations about the future affect immediate needs.

2   Deal with the way the patient actually is. Look for small signs of progress.

3   Ask professionals to share information. Sit in on rehabilitation or assessment sessions; ask for and read assessment reports. Professionals should be more than happy to include as many members of the family as possible.

4   Recognize that you need to work through a series of emotions, including anger, guilt and grief, but cannot if you pretend that everything will be all right.

5   Acceptance of reality takes time. It is only when the family have come to terms with reality that they can help the person with the head injury to accept their new life ahead.

ANGER AND FRUSTRATION

Examples

1   A father refuses to co-operate with police investigations.

2   A mother becomes irate because the nurse only spent 30 minutes attempting to get her daughter to eat lunch.

3   A wife is angry with her husband (the patient) for being slow, and for not appreciating all the trauma that she has been through.

4   A mother screams and yells at her daughter, who has forgotten to do the dishes after being told three times.

5   A wife and carer explodes in anger at a relative who is critical of the way she manages her husband, saying, "You just don't know what it's like because you don't live here, so keep your stupid comments to yourself."

Understanding Anger and Frustration

Anger is a natural emotion to feel in the circumstances. However anger about what has happened is often directed at a variety of individuals, including doctors, nurses, family members, God, and patients themselves. A second aspect of anger is to do with frustration. If you are a person who is used to 'being in control', the occurrence of a head injury in a family can be the most frustrating event of your life. Recovery does not follow a smooth pattern and definite answers are difficult to find. It is difficult to plan anything and now life is riddled with uncertainty. What makes the situation worse is that often people outside the immediate family do not understand the deeper problem and sometimes can be insensitive with their comments.

Coping with Anger and Frustration

1   Recognize that you are primarily angry about what has happened. Apologize ahead of time.

2   Identify the triggers for anger, for example a particular nurse, a friend of the patient's, a critical relative. Avoid if possible.

3   Express your anger. Ventilate it with someone you trust. Don't let it eat you away. Seek counselling if necessary.

4   Discharge some of the anger in a vigorous, productive, physical activity (sport, house cleaning, walking or starting a self-help group).

GUILT

Examples

1   A parent thinks, "If only I hadn't bought him that motorcycle for his birthday", and blames himself for the accident.

2   A wife thinks, "It would have been better if he had died." Then she feels terribly guilty.

3   A mother feels guilty taking time off for herself and enjoying herself, thinking, "I should be at my daughter's bedside."

4   A mother feels guilty about refusing the unreasonable demands of the patient and allows her to do just as she pleases.

5   A wife thinks, "Why me?" and feels resentful that all this has happened. Afterwards she feels guilty.

Understanding Guilt

If you are the type of person who has taken on guilt before, you will be easily trapped into taking on mountains of it if a member of your family has a head injury. The circumstances of a head injury provide multiple opportunities for feeling that you have not done your best for yourself, the patient, other family members and others concerned. Beware of the little voice in your head saying things like: "I should have", "I ought to", "I must", because these statements will make you feel worse, and will not help the situation. When you notice yourself using the words 'should', 'ought' and 'must', try challenging those statements by asking yourself the question, "Why should I?" or "How could I?" Guilt is the result of an individual feeling overly responsible for somebody else.

Coping with Guilt

1   Accept guilt as a normal feeling over which we have minimal control.

2   Don't expect yourself to be perfect. You can be angry, tearful, blaming, sad and critical. Accept how you feel. After months of caring for a difficult, unrewarding patient it is natural at times to 'wish he were dead'.

3   Accept that you are not responsible. Sometimes these things happen. No amount of taking the blame will alter what has happened.

4   Schedule your guilt session. For example, agree to worry only between 8 o'clock and 9 o'clock, and then make an effort to forget it for the rest of the day.

5   Try to distract yourself with some engrossing activity, such as gardening or sport.

6   Accept that there may be little you can do to change your loved one,

so there is no need to feel guilty when you see no improvement. Allow yourself to let go, take care of yourself and rejoin the human race.

GRIEF AND DEPRESSION

Examples

1   A tearful mother realizes that, after months of rehabilitation, her son with a head injury will not be going to university.

2   A wife realizes that the strong, dominant, loving man whom she married has gone, and will not return. She feels depressed and lonely.

3   After discharge from the hospital services, the family realizes that the problems for the person with a head injury are long-term. Life will never be the same.

4   Family members shed tears looking at old holiday photographs of happy times.

Understanding Grief and Depression

After a certain point in the process of rehabilitation, progress will slow down; a plateau will be reached. It is often at this point that members of the family realize that life will never return to the way it was, expectations have to alter and plans have to be changed. It is a time to recognize the enormous losses that have occurred. Families need to grieve for those losses: the injury has taken so many things away, even though they have not physically lost the family member. This grief and sadness is often delayed, because the family has been so busy they have not had the opportunity to grieve. It is important to recognize that this sadness is a stage that everybody needs to go through before reaching a point of acceptance. Feeling sad or depressed, although painful, is a sign of progress, rather than something to worry about and try to avoid.

Most family members will experience grief at some point, particularly if they have been very close to the patient, or if they now feel hopelessly trapped. Symptoms may include anxiety attacks, disturbed sleep and eating habits, obsessive thoughts, lethargy and agitation. The overriding feeling is that of helplessness and hopelessness. This reaction is just as natural and predictable as it is for the bereaved to mourn.

Coping with Grief and Depression

1   Allow yourself to cry. Allow yourself to remember and talk about the past. Have a good cry over old photographs.

2   Accept that the past is behind you and that the future will be different.

3   Modify your goals and expectations. Very few people who have had severe head injury return to their former level of functioning, but that does not mean that they cannot be happy at another level.

4   Make the most of what the person with the head injury can do, and try to forget the things that they can't.

5   If you feel that you are 'emotionally stuck', seek professional help. It may be that you are feeling so numb you cannot feel sadness or grief. Perhaps you are feeling suicidal. If you are using alcohol and drugs to dull your misery, you may need to deal with the feelings directly so that you can move on.

TIREDNESS

Examples

1   Parents sit up at night with their son who has a head injury until 2 am.

2 A mother finds it difficult to sleep at night because of worrying. Her attempts to nap during the day are fruitless because of racing thoughts.

3 A wife with children, who has to work and visit the hospital, as well as carrying out all the jobs that her husband normally did, feels completely exhausted at the end of every day.

4 A mother reports that looking after her demanding, 20-year-old, head-injured son is more tiring than looking after him when he was a baby.

5 "My husband is such hard work; he talks non-stop. At the end of the day I'm exhausted."

Understanding Tiredness

Having a relative involved in a head injury creates a long-standing trauma. The emotional upheavals and physical tension are in themselves tiring. Loss of sleep through worry, and being incredibly busy travelling to and from hospital, means that the relative is usually experiencing debilitating tiredness and fatigue. Often the idea of looking after yourself, through food, diet or exercise, is rarely considered. In some ways it is analogous to having a new-born baby, but it is much worse.

Coping with Tiredness

1 Look after yourself. Eat well and try to get as much sleep as possible. You are no good to your loved ones if you are ill.

2 Put off until tomorrow what is not absolutely necessary.

3 Delegate responsibility. Ask friends and family to do things. Others are often only too pleased to help.

4 Do not feel that you have to be constantly by the patient's side.

5 Learn relaxation exercises if you have difficulty sleeping.

LOSS OF LOVE

Examples

1 A wife says, "He used to be strong, active, loving and affectionate. We used to laugh, but now he's completely wrapped up in his own problems and gives me little or no affection."

2 A wife says, "I could always rely on him, I felt safe in his arms. Now he needs me and I'm the one that has to cuddle him."

3 Parents bemoan the fact that, even four years after the injury, it is still them 'giving' to their daughter and getting little back in return, in terms of affection or appreciation.

4 A wife says, "I feel that I'm married to a stranger. He is not the man I once loved."

5 A husband says, "She never touches or cuddles me any more and she's lost all interest in sex."

Understanding Loss of Love

A head injury can affect a person's emotional responding, libido, sensitivity, ability to empathize, and also encourage a tendency towards self-centredness. This will invariably mean that the spouse, parent or child of a person with a head injury will notice a change in the fabric of their relationship; it means they will get less love. This is often more difficult for a spouse than for a parent or child. We all choose our partners because of their personalities; we do not choose our parents or children. Often it is easier for a mother to look after her adult son because he is returning to a childlike dependent state; she has her son back.

It is often recorded that a wife will say that she still loves her husband but feels that their love has changed, and is no longer the romantic love that first attracted her to him, but more akin to the love between sister and brother.

Coping with Loss of Love

1   Talk to the loved one the way you used to.

2   Let the loved one make as many decisions as possible or ask their opinion, even if it is not necessarily needed.

3   Approach the situation as you would a new relationship.

LACK OF TIME FOR SELF

Examples

1   A wife does not go out with friends because she feels that she ought to look after her husband who has had a head injury.

2   A mother has left her job and gives up all outside contacts to look after her head-injured son. In reality, her son does not need or want her around all the time.

3   A family insists that they have to be with their daughter 24 hours a day. Family members are unwilling to take any risk regarding leaving her on her own.

4   A sociable family stopped having guests around because of their head-injured son's embarrassing behaviour. The teenage daughter stopped asking her friends around because her brother 'could not keep his hands to himself'.

5   A head-injured husband demands that his wife stay with him all the time.

Understanding Lack of Time for Self

It is understandable that, initially, when the person with the head injury returns home, the family is supportive and inward looking. It is only natural that at first they are busy adjusting and have less time for outside interests and friends. However the danger is that this habit becomes long-standing and difficult to break. It is a mistake to isolate oneself from old contacts. It is possible that many old friendships may dwindle because the family feels that these old friends do not understand, cannot accept the problems, or feel uncomfortable. If this happens make every effort to form new acquaintances. Be firm with yourself and recognize that you have needs too; set boundaries and learn to say 'no' to the person with the head injury. Make time for yourself.

Coping with Lack of Time for Self

1   Try to avoid setting up a pattern of decreased social contact.

2   Do not give up your job unless this is absolutely necessary.

3   Do not convince yourself that your care is indispensable. You must recognize and give time to your own needs. If you do not you will wear yourself out and be no good to anybody.

4   Plan social activities, giving them priority. Try to talk about things other than the person with the head injury.

5   Both carer and cared-for need to have some time on their own. This may mean altering the layout of your house, or letting a friend look after the person with the injury for part of the day, or letting them go away for respite care for a week or two. Learn to let go!

ROLE CHANGES

Examples

1 "Mark always did everything. He looked after all the household bills, the car, money, shopping, repairs, in short, everything. I suppose he was like a father figure. Since his accident he can't do all those things. The tables have turned. It took me a long time to accept it. I used to feel really angry with him and still do. But it has certainly made me stand on my own two feet. I'm a much stronger, more capable person because of it."

2 "All our lives we always thought Mum could do everything. If there was a problem in the family, my brothers and sisters, aunts and I would always turn to Mum. She was involved in everything that was going on. Now we all have to hold back. Even though she looks well she just can't cope with other people's problems in the way she used to."

3 "My relationship with my elder brother has changed. Sometimes I feel that I'm the elder brother, but in other areas he still is."

4 "It took me five years to truly accept the personality changes and to totally convince myself that I could handle this new person."

5 "Since Dad's accident he's changed. I have to be much more careful and quiet, because he gets angry a lot quicker."

Understanding Role Changes

We all play a variety of different roles or have well established habits within our family, our work and our social life. These might include being breadwinner, decision maker, joker, helper, trouble maker, dependant and problem solver. Changes produced by head injury often mean that our roles have to change: the breadwinner becomes unemployed; the leader and organizer now needs to be led and organized; the father figure may take on a role closer to dependent child; the life and soul of the party becomes withdrawn and lacking in confidence. However, because the roles of the person with a head injury change, so do the roles of other family members. In a marriage, if the husband with a head injury can no longer deal with the family's finances and bill paying, the wife has to do it herself; her role changes as well. In some cases she may have to pay bills for the first time, become better organized and make important decisions on her own for the first time in her life. This requires the ability to change. Inevitably, initially this 'having to change' produces many feelings of fear, anger, resentment and frustration. The family member may say, "Why should I?", "Why me?" This is a normal reaction. However, if these negative feelings can be overcome, the relative or spouse of the head-injured person has an opportunity to change and grow into a stronger, more fully rounded, capable person.

Coping with Role Changes

1   Discuss changes openly with family and friends. Identify areas where there may be difficulties and ask for help.

2   Recognize that you may have to take responsibility in implementing these changes, as the person with the head injury will probably see himself as he was before the accident.

3   Try to express your feelings about these changes. Don't store up resentment.

4   Try to view change as a challenge and an opportunity rather than a problem.

OVER-PROTECTIVENESS

Examples

1   A father says, "Simon can't be left on his own for one minute of the day. He's a danger to himself and other people."

2   A mother says, "We make all the decisions for Colin these days, right down to the wallpaper and posters to put on his bedroom wall."

3   A mother says, "My son has a drink problem now, as an indirect result of his head injury, so we dare not let him go out on his own in case he is tempted to go into a pub. So I just go everywhere with him."

4   A mother cooks, feeds, shops, cleans and washes for her son, even though with some effort he could do these things for himself.

Understanding Over-protectiveness

Over-protectiveness is particularly common when patients are discharged to parents' homes. This is understandable initially, as the person may be very fragile, dependent and needy at first. However, with encouragement, the person with the head injury becomes more independent and as this happens the family needs to withdraw. Rather than doing things for him, family members need to help him do things for himself. The more families do for the person with the injury, the less will be the improvement. Often this over-protectiveness happens because the family members feel sorry, guilty or worried about a possible second injury. Family members need to ask themselves, "Is this the best thing to do for him in the long run?" The person with the head injury needs the opportunity to test his skills, and either succeed or fail in as normal a way as possible. If family members are continually over-protective, the message that they are subtly conveying to their loved one is, "You are incompetent, inadequate and untrustworthy." This can easily undermine already fragile self-esteem and confidence. Also, as time goes by, the person with the injury feels resentful and angry at the relative who is "always doing things for me". The family should try to recognize the need to be firm and to take some calculated risks. After all, risk is inherent in everything we do. We all need the dignity and opportunity of risk to be fully human. This applies equally to people with a head injury.

Coping with Over-protectiveness

1   Recognize your over-protective tendencies. Ask yourself what else the person with the head injury could possibly do without help. Ask for an outside opinion if you feel that you are too close to the subject.

2   Understand and recognize the feelings behind your over-protectiveness. Especially consider the possibility of guilt. Talk it over with someone — a friend, social worker, counsellor or psychologist.

3   Acknowledge the individual's limitations but focus on his strengths. Monitor gradual step-by-step progress.

4   Accept that, in order to make progress, you need to take some risks. This may involve letting the person travel alone, cook a meal or be left alone in the house. There is always a chance that he will get lost, or burn a saucepan, but these risks need to be taken if real progress is to be made.

UNDER-PROTECTIVENESS

Examples

1   "My wife says that she can't remember things, but she's all right really. Everyone on her side of the family has a bad memory."

2   "I insisted that Neil should come away with the lads for the weekend because I really thought it would do him good. Saturday night he

claimed to be exhausted, and spent the rest of the weekend sleeping in the back of the van."

3 "He had all weekend to decorate our bedroom and he still hasn't finished."

4 "Mother has always liked to be busy. She complains more since the accident, but I don't think she's different now from how she was before."

Understanding Under-protectiveness

In situations where there is under-protectiveness, family and relatives are often still at the level of denial of the disability, expecting the person with the head injury to be as absolutely capable as before. There has been no redefining of roles, and the husband, wife, mother, father or schoolchild is expected to carry on as before. This often creates anger and resentment because the person cannot do it, and fails to live up to false expectations. The family or friends have not moved to the level of realistic acceptance. It is very difficult to accept that all family members' lives have got to change.

Coping with Under-protectiveness

1 There is an enormous need to communicate and exchange information concerning changed roles.

2 The person with the head injury needs to be assertive and learn to say, 'No', or 'I have difficulty doing that. Could you help me?'

3 Seek professional help. A third party with experience of head injury can provide information which allows everybody to be realistic. Encourage family and friends to look at professional reports and assessments.

4 Recognize your feelings of reluctance to accept the changed role.

5   Allow the person with the head injury to make a few small mistakes, but not too many, so that they lose confidence and dignity.

6   Recognize that things need to be different. Try to create a regular, consistent, stable environment.

Mark's Story

"I recognize that I've always been a 'driven' character who has spent his life doing 101 things at the same time. I've always looked after Fiona (my wife), earning the money, paying the bills, servicing the cars, repairing the house, organizing holidays and weekends, even doing the shopping. Since my accident I just can't do it all, but she still expects the same from me. When I was discharged from hospital after two weeks, she'd moved out of our house back to her parents, because the toilet system had broken. Why she couldn't have just rung a plumber I don't know! It's so difficult because I feel angry with her for being so inadequate and I know she feels angry with me. I feel that I've always been there for her, helping and protecting her, but now, for once, I need her help and she's not there. I recognize that we've got to readjust the balance of our relationship. I can't go on being this father figure doing everything and she can't go on being the little child." ■

A Wife's Story

"We had been married for seven years and had two small children when Frank had his accident. He was in a coma for a week. I remember being elated when they said he was going to live, and felt that he would be back to normal in a few weeks. I was wrong. Although in the years since his injury Frank has made a good recovery, he is different from the way he was. Before the accident he was full of energy and life, always joking, brimming with exciting ideas and plans. We would go away camping at weekends and frequently entertain friends and family. Now Frank has little enthusiasm, is slower, has lost his sense of fun, gets very irritable, and is often preoccupied by his problems. I miss his friendship, intimacy, partnership and the sexual relationship that we had. I still love Frank but in a different way, almost like an elder sister. Life is much harder now because not only do I have to look after the two children but I have to keep an eye on Frank. I know the eldest boy misses how his dad used to be, but both children have accepted things.

There are no pretty solutions; I know he won't suddenly get better. I must say at times I have wondered whether a separation would be the best thing, especially when Frank loses his temper with the kids. I feel angry and think it's just not fair, but then we settle down again and I know that I just couldn't leave him. I'm lucky because my family live close by and help out, and we did get a good settlement, so money is not a problem. I wish Frank's family could be more realistic; they still don't accept that he's changed and close their eyes to our real problems — that irritates me. I do still feel angry at the lack of help we received when Frank was discharged from hospital, and the total ignorance of most people about the real problems of head injury.

I've always been reasonably realistic and would say to anybody in my position that you need stamina, resilience and commitment. You also need to alter your dreams, hopes, goals and expectations. The possibility of divorce or a separation are very real and I think it helps to openly discuss these issues. I still miss 'the old Frank', and still get that feeling of emptiness, but we keep going, for better or for worse, and we do have our occasional sweet moments." ■

SPECIAL ISSUES

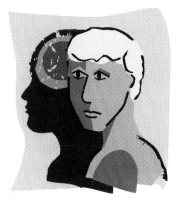

Chapter 8

RETURNING TO WORK

Most people who have received a head injury regard a return to work as a very important goal to aim towards. However, especially in the case of people with a severe injury, the long-term work prospects are disappointing. Research suggests that only approximately 19–29 per cent of those who had a job before suffering a severe head injury are back at work, either full- or part-time, five years after injury. These figures may well disguise the fact that a number of people are in situations of sheltered or protected employment with a sympathetic employer or organization. The person's return to work after a head injury, and the extent of the difficulties he encounters, depend on several factors, such as the severity of the injury, his array of residual long-term side-effects, the type of occupation, the amount of vocational rehabilitation he receives and how he approaches the task of returning to work.

Experts suggest that people who have had a period of post-traumatic amnesia (PTA) of between 1-14 days might be able to return to the same job, but be less capable. A period of PTA of between 2-4 weeks means that there will be definite difficulties, which will make it unlikely that the person will be able to perform the same job. A PTA of between 4-12 weeks suggests that the person will be lucky to get part-time employment, while a PTA of over 12 weeks suggests that the person is likely to be unemployed, or work in a sheltered environment, or do voluntary work.

Certain groups tend to have special problems. The executive or manager, who has reached his position because of his ability to analyse, organize, plan, solve problems and make decisions, has difficulty because these much-needed, aptly named, 'executive functions' are the very skills which are often impaired. The 'above-average student' has difficulties because often marginal impairments reduce performance down towards the average range. This is often a shattering blow and is further exacerbated by the fact that he will have to work much harder to learn things which previously were easily learned. The 'below-average student' also may have special problems, as teachers and parents may not recognize new subtle memory and attention problems, but instead will attribute these problems to the fact that 'he always had difficulties at school'. Self-employed people, with limited insurance, also have special problems, as they feel that they cannot stay off work for too long — otherwise their business will suffer. There is no absolute, right way to approach returning to work, but there are a number of sensible pointers which can act as guidelines.

Be positive and realistic Thinking positively does not just mean saying, "I will go back to work", but rather it means carefully considering and planning the best options. It means saying, "What can I do?" and also "What am I going to have difficulty with?" A useful exercise might be to draw up a list of work activities and rate performance before and after injury. It is very important for the head-injured person to rate himself on this list. The list must include all aspects of work. A few examples include using machines, manual work, remembering facts, figure work, attending meetings, driving, making decisions, organizing ideas and thoughts, dealing with correspondence, using the telephone and standing for long periods.

In one study it was found that the most important predictor of whether a person would successfully return to work was not severity of injury as measured by duration of coma, or even cognitive functioning, but rather, realistic acceptance of the disability and acceptance of self. Those at peace with themselves have a greater chance of returning to work.

Recognize the common problems It is important to recognize the common problems which can interfere with performance at work. These are:

(a) poor memory — which means slow learning;
(b) poor concentration — which means easy distractability;
(c) slowed thinking — difficulty understanding fast, complex speech or ideas;
(d) executive difficulties — difficulty organizing, planning, analysing,

making decisions, judgement, and using initiative;

(e) tiredness;

(f) lowered tolerance of frustration — easily becoming upset, difficulty coping with stress, difficulty working to deadlines;

(g) poor insight — lack of awareness of these difficulties;

(h) unrealistic expectations — lack of acceptance of disability and self;

(i) impaired interpersonal skills.

Return at the right time There is an almost inevitable tendency for the person with the head injury to attempt to return to work too early. Because a good physical recovery has been made, people assume a similar cognitive recovery. At the same time the person with the injury invariably over-estimates his own ability. This very often results in a premature return to work, creating difficulties and then failure. Returning to work too early and failing can have a positive and a negative effect. The positive effect is that it often increases insight and awareness and helps the person to readjust their expectations to a more realistic level. The negative effect is that it can severely dent the person's confidence and produce feelings of depression and demoralization. This fine balance between improving insight and the negative effect on confidence needs to be carefully considered.

Start small It is better to start on a part-time basis if possible, beginning with as little as two–three hours for two–three days a week, and then work up slowly. It is important not to take on too much. It is often a good idea to start with a sheltered work placement, or to carry out some voluntary work to test strengths and weaknesses.

Educate the employer Employers simply do not understand the subtle, hidden, long-term side-effects of head injury. Like everybody else, they view disability in physical terms, expecting a wheelchair or a stick. If they do not understand they will usually reach faulty conclusions, thinking, "He's just lazy" or "He's malingering." The employer can be helped to understand if he is provided with information. This will prepare him for the fact that there will be difficulties, which can be overcome if they are anticipated.

Look for a job with a high degree of structure, consistency and familiarity This means that the job has a regular routine, rather than having constant changes and disruptions. Look to establish a well stamped in, regular pattern of behaviour. Tasks need to be quite specific and unambiguous. At first it is probably best if the work does not require a great deal of planning, analysis and organizational skills. A structured job does not necessarily have to be a boring, repetitive job. If possible, look for a job that taps old, well learned, unimpaired skills, rather than a job that requires a great deal of new learning.

Find a work environment with few distractions and interruptions Beware of environments where there is a great deal of background noise or commotion, or a high degree of chaotic stimulation, as this often makes concentrating on a particular task difficult. Filtering out unwanted distractions is often difficult after a head injury.

Break the job down into small skills The job becomes more manageable if broken down into a number of smaller skills or building-blocks. Make a list of all the skills needed to do the job. Once skills have been broken down into small units and described they can be understood and learned more easily in a step-by-step approach.

Use compensatory strategies This means using any external aids to help memory, concentration and organizational ability. It is helpful to use lists, diaries, charts on the wall, tape recorders, labels and so on. It is better to plan important meetings early in the day if tiredness is a problem.

Arrange for careful monitoring and feedback The person with the injury is not always the best person to judge how he is doing. It helps to have somebody else monitoring progress, identifying problems and giving feedback about strengths and weaknesses. An idea which has worked well for some people with a head injury is to have a colleague or workmate act as a 'mentor' or 'work coach' for a short while following the return to work. It is better to anticipate and expect difficulties, and then treat them as challenges. The person who thinks that they will have no problems is more likely to fail.

Three Examples of Successful Return to Work after Severe Head Injury

Paul had just completed his PhD on computer-based models of weather forecasting and was considered a 'fast track' high-flyer by the meteorological office. Tragically he was involved in a climbing accident, which resulted in his being in a coma for two weeks, leaving him with a severe head injury. He made a good physical recovery and following intensive rehabilitation returned to work part-time after 12 months. He found the work difficult because of his poor memory and slowed thinking processes. Physically he looked very well and colleagues' expectations were unrealistically high. Their expectations were made even higher and more unrealistic when Paul talked about his previous work on his PhD. On the one hand, he could remember most of the highly complex theoretical work, which he had learned before his accident, but, on the other hand, he could not remember the simple instructions to work the new computer system. When he spoke about his PhD, people commented on how brilliant he was; however they failed to take into account that Paul had great difficulty remembering and learning even the simplest new information. He struggled on bravely for 18 months, before being moved into easier, more comfortable areas of work. Work was still stressful because people did not understand his particular difficulties. Eventually Paul reduced his hours of paid employment and worked part-time at a much lower grade, spending the rest of his time working in a Headway day centre.

Stephen returned to work as a carpet fitter eight months after a severe head injury. He thought he had prepared himself well, engaging in a rigorous fitness training programme. Unfortunately he had to stop work after three days because of difficulties with organizing, planning, memory and tiredness. Stephen became depressed and made an unsuccessful suicide attempt. After another four months of 'sulking around the house' he acquired another job with a different firm. Again he had difficulties, and was made redundant after just five weeks. This time he lost a great deal of confidence, became seriously depressed and made another attempt on his life. He was admitted to a psychiatric hospital, where he stayed for two months. It took a long time for Stephen to regain his confidence and return to work again. It is now three years since his accident and he has worked regularly as a self-employed carpet fitter for the last six months. He recognizes that his standard of work is very slightly lower than before, but he still sees himself as being better than most. He is now happy and settled and looks back on those first two years after his injury as a 'nightmare' of raised and dashed expectations. He also acknowledges that he had tried to return to work too early.

Jenny returned to her job as an accountant for a group of farmers, nine months after her accident. She started off slowly but the work piled up and she had dreadful difficulty. She said, "I would make mistakes with the easiest calculations, I'd forget to sign letters, or put them in the wrong envelope, I'd forget what I'd said in a conversation. I would put things away very safely in the most sensible place, then later would spend ridiculous amounts of time looking for them. It was hard meeting new people as, apart from the difficulty of finding words to make sensible sentences, and remembering what I'd said, I just didn't feel the same person. I'd get these terrible headaches where I would just have to go home. It got bad because other people were having to do my work and I felt dreadfully guilty. I'd cry if people said even the slightest thing that was nasty. After great, protracted negotiation and 18 months of sheer misery I took early retirement on the grounds of ill health. I now have a simple, less demanding part-time job, as a doctor's receptionist, and I actually enjoy it."

All three examples illustrate the difficulties of returning to work after head injury. The three people all experienced emotional and practical problems and ended up working in an altered capacity or different situation. Encouragingly all three are still employed and are enjoying their work.

CHILDREN WITH HEAD INJURY

It is estimated that for every 30 newborn children one will have a significant brain injury before reaching driving age. After the grouping of young men between the ages of 17 and 30, children are the second most likely group to sustain head injury. As would be expected, in this age group there is a higher proportion of domestic accidents than in other age groups, particularly falls from windows, playground equipment and down the stairs. Proportionally there is a smaller number of road traffic accidents involving children, although a higher rate of pedestrian accidents, because children are not as safe and aware of road safety as adults. Therefore there is a relatively smaller number of severe head injuries in children, as compared to mild or moderate injuries. It is estimated that at least 10 per cent of head injuries in children under the age of five years are due to 'non-accidental injury' or child abuse; of particular significance is the so-called 'shaken baby syndrome'. The baby may have a significant brain injury without suffering any damage to the skull.

Cerebral Plasticity in Children

The difference between head injuries in adults and children is that an injury to a child occurs in the context of continuing development and an incomplete repertoire of abilities. The child's brain is still evolving and organizing itself in a very complex way. Scientists talk about 'cerebral plasticity' in children, which means the brain is gradually organizing itself and has not 'set' in an irreversible or immutable way. After a certain age, probably around 10 years, the brain settles down and particular areas develop specialist functions. There are many examples of very young children having major brain surgery because of epilepsy (hemispherectomy) where half the brain is removed. In most cases it is the left hemisphere which is removed. The result is that the epileptic seizures stop, and the right hemisphere takes over most of the functions normally associated with the absent left hemisphere, such as language skills. The individual will often have some intellectual limitations, but cases have been reported where the child has gone on to acquire a university degree. These examples demonstrate cerebral plasticity, and how the brain can rearrange itself, particularly if injured very early on.

One famous neuropsychologist once stated, "If I'm going to have a brain injury, I'd best have it earlier rather than later in life." This somewhat glib remark reflects the general notion that there is more adaptability to serious head injury in the developing nervous system than there is at maturity. However, more recently it has been recognized that the extent of cerebral plasticity in children was perhaps exaggerated in the past, and children still have an extremely difficult time after brain injury. Let us examine some of the particular problems that children have.

Particular Problems with Children

Significant effects of head injury in children can often be overlooked or forgotten, for a number of reasons. Firstly, children have much greater difficulty expressing themselves, as their vocabulary is limited. It is more difficult for a seven-year-old to say, "I've got a headache", "I find I'm forgetting things", or "I can't concentrate." Secondly, because children are still growing up, developing and changing over time, it is difficult to know what to compare their abilities with. It is more difficult for a child than an adult to say, "I used to be able to do that but now I can't." An adult has years of past experience with which to compare a skill, such as memory or concentration. It is also quite common for the residual effects of a head injury to be forgotten by parents and teachers, who may say, "But the accident was years ago. He must have recovered by now." The child is in no position to stand up and say, "I am still affected by the accident", whereas an adult would be able to recognize and articulate such an effect.

The two main problem areas for children are often behavioural self-control and academic performance at school. After head injury the individual may become more impulsive, disinhibited, outspoken, restless, careless, aggressive, less in control of his behaviour, irritable or emotional. Significantly, children spend the majority of their childhood gradually learning the necessary skills to control their behaviour. A head injury can often severely affect or set back that gradual process, so the child returns to the pre-school stage of temper tantrums. It is often noted that behaviour becomes worse when the child is tired. Three possible strategies might possibly help: (1) encourage physical activity to work off that irritability and restlessness; (2) give the child plenty of sleep and rest; and (3) recognize the difficulties, accept that they may be due to the injury and recognize that in these circumstances parents need to be firm from an early stage.

The question of when or whether the child should return to school is always difficult. A careful balance has to be struck between the need for the child to have contact with his peers, and being sure that the child has recovered sufficiently to be able to cope with the school environment. It is difficult to imagine a more stressful environment to which to return after a head injury than that of school. School represents a set of very stressful situations involving new learning and multiple demands to pay attention, remember information and to exercise self-control. If somebody has an impaired memory, poor attention and is mentally and physically slower than they were, they are going to have difficulties. They may have already missed a large chunk of work which needs catching up. This will further exacerbate the problem. It is not surprising that children who have had a head injury fall behind academically and find that they cannot cope. Very often this decline in achievements may not become obvious for some time. Teacher assessments and examinations are a relatively insensitive measure to assess these subtle difficulties. Very often the child's behaviour deteriorates and they become labelled as 'naughty troublemakers'. This disruptive maladaptive behaviour is often the only way children can cope with their predicament and is a way of diverting attention away from true performance difficulties.

It is important for parents to let the school know about the injury, alert the form teacher, and try to explain about the difficulties. But, of course, there is no guarantee that they will be understood. A gradual return to school, starting off with a couple of hours and working upwards to a full day, is also important. This allows time to increase mental and physical stamina. If a cognitive assessment by a psychologist has not already been carried out, and you are concerned, ask the school to request an assessment by an educational psychologist or clinical psychologist with knowledge of brain injury. If necessary, this information can be put together in a 'statement of educational needs' and special support or teaching can be provided.

Practical Steps for Teachers

- Establish good communication between parents and school and between the teachers of the pupil with a head injury.

- Establish planned regular meetings between parents and school and other agencies to monitor the situation.

- Look at information about head injury. Understand more about the cognitive, emotional and behavioural problems that follow injury.

- Consider making modifications to the pupil's timetable.

- Ensure that the pupil is paying attention when important things are said.

- Present homework tasks explicitly, checking that they are written correctly and understood.

- Allow sufficient time for task completion.

- Monitor progress more frequently and provide additional help if necessary. Give extra encouragement.

- Check and deal with bullying and teasing. Help classmates to understand what has happened.

- Make special arrangements for examinations.

CLAIMING COMPENSATION

Contacting a Solicitor

Contact a solicitor as soon as possible after the accident. Choose a solicitor who specializes in personal injury claims and has experience of head injury. You can find the names of such a specialist from a number of sources: (a) Headway National Head Injuries Association has a list of experienced solicitors; (b) the Law Society will recommend two or three solicitors in your area; there is also a new specialist section, The Association of Personal Injury Lawyers; (c) your local Headway group.

Do not be afraid of asking the solicitor about his experience in personal injury work. If he has little or no experience of head injury it might be wise to find somebody else. Remember, the sooner you contact a solicitor the better. Claims must be made within three years of the injury. Keep a diary of all expenses incurred from day one! At a later date someone will ask about transport costs, loss of earnings and so on.

Counter-productive Thoughts about Seeking Compensation

We haven't got a case; it was our fault

Many people fail to claim compensation simply because they are not aware of their legal rights. They think the accident was their own fault, or they are not entitled to a claim. In a recent survey of 37 injured people, who all thought the accident was their own fault, 11 of these accidents could have been caused wholly or partially by the negligence of some other party.

I couldn't stand going to court

Don't be put off by the idea of going to court. Statistics indicate that only 2 per cent of personal injury cases actually reach court, and half of these are settled 'at the door of the court' by agreement, without evidence being given to the judge.

We can't afford the legal fees

Don't be put off by fear of legal fees. Experienced solicitors understand that accident victims often have no income or capital. Initial legal advice is often available free of charge or at a very low cost. Thereafter an application can be made for Legal Aid. Your Citizen's Advice Bureau or Voluntary Law Surgery will give you advice about the various legal aid schemes. If you are successful, the other side's insurers will be ordered to pay all legal aid costs.

We can't claim against him because he's family

It is important to note that a family member injured as a passenger in a car accident can claim against the driver, even if he is a member of the same family. So a child injured can claim against the parent's insurance. Do not be put off; most of the dealings are at the level of solicitors and insurance companies.

What Your Solicitor Will Do

Making the claim

A good solicitor is like a non-playing captain, since it is his job to make the claim and then to pull together a team of specialists who will make reports to support that claim. In the majority of cases in the English legal system it is necessary to identify somebody whose negligence caused the accident. You, or the injured party, are then referred to as the 'plaintiff', and the people who supposedly caused the accident as the 'defendant'. Your solicitor will write a letter of claim at an early stage to the defendant, who will then pass it on to their insurers. Your solicitor will then correspond with the insurance company to find out whether they will contest the claim or whether they admit liability, and how much damages they will pay. If the insurers will not admit liability, your solicitor should take steps to issue court proceedings on your behalf.

Obtaining evidence relating to liability

Your solicitor should interview all relevant witnesses and obtain signed statements from them. If it was a road traffic accident, he should obtain a copy of the police report. This will give information about position of vehicles and weather conditions, and statements. If the police have not prosecuted anybody, it usually means that the evidence is not strong enough to obtain a criminal conviction 'beyond reasonable doubt'. This does not mean that you cannot make a civil claim. Indeed the vast majority of civil claims succeed despite the absence of any criminal conviction.

Obtaining expert medical and professional reports

Your solicitor will arrange for expert medical and professional reports to be prepared describing the injuries sustained. The injured party may have to attend an examination and it is a good idea to be accompanied by a friend or relative, who can describe how the life of the head-injured person has been affected by the accident. The insurance company acting for the other side, the defendant, may also request separate examinations. Your solicitor should be asking for a number of specialist reports from any of the following professionals:

(a) The attending physician/surgeon in whose care the patient was at the time of admission, who can describe the nature and severity of the injuries.

(b) A neurosurgeon, if one has been involved.

(c) Members of other medical specialities, depending on the injuries, such as an orthopaedic surgeon or a plastic surgeon.

(d) A consultant in rehabilitation to give a medical overview.

(e) A clinical neuropsychologist with special interest in head injury to carry out tests of intellectual ability, memory, concentration and personality, and to offer insight into long-term prospects.

Other reports may include those from a speech therapist, an occupational therapist, a physiotherapist, a psychiatrist, a case manager, an architect and others.

Working out the claim

Working out the claim is a specialist job and often the solicitor will employ a specialist accountant. Basically a claim for damages is made up of two elements, 'special damages' and 'general damages'. *Special damages* are awarded to compensate for a direct financial loss incurred as a result of the accident: for example, loss of wages, private medical fees, the cost of equipment, travelling expenses and damage to vehicle or clothing. *General damages* include pain and suffering, the loss of capacity due to the physical and mental symptoms and disabilities, future losses such as loss of earnings or promotion prospects, the cost of providing personal care, the cost of special accommodation, the cost of physiotherapy, speech therapy and other specialist therapies, and the cost of aids, equipment and transport. Beginning as soon as possible after the accident, it is a good idea to keep a record of all additional expenses and to retain receipts. It is also useful to keep a record or diary of pain and suffering.

Obtaining an interim payment if possible

An interim payment means the other side paying some of the damages immediately or well before the case is settled. It has been said that 'interim payments are the life blood for a head-injured person', because the money is needed for rehabilitation immediately, which is better than in four years' time. Your solicitor should always consider this option, especially if your case is a strong one, such as if you were injured as a passenger. This money can help to pay for specialist medical, therapeutic and residential treatments and will improve recovery prospects and reduce dependence, thereby reducing the final settlement. It is thus to the benefit of the defendant's insurers to make interim payment because it means that the patient will get maximum rehabilitation, become more independent, and hence the ultimate damages will be less.

The Settlement

Court proceedings

Once your solicitor has collected together sufficient evidence he will instruct a barrister to prepare a statement of claims. This is a document which sets out the essential facts and the legal basis for your claim. This document is served upon the defendant or his solicitor and they will prepare a defence which should say whether liability will be admitted or contested. After this exchange of information, your solicitor will set the case down for trial. Your solicitor will ensure that all relevant documents, plans and photographs are filed at the court. Quite often the other side will make some final effort to settle the claim before the case is heard in court and, as stated earlier, settlements are frequently reached at the door of the court.

If the insurers accept that the defendant is legally liable for the plaintiff's injuries then the only issue is the amount of damages you will recover. Sometimes the insurer will accept liability, provided that you agree to a deduction for 'contributory negligence'. For example, if the injured person was not wearing a crash helmet or a seat belt the insurers may wish to reduce your claim by 25 per cent.

Structured settlements

Many solicitors, barristers and judges believe that a structured settlement is preferable to a single lump sum. The injured person would receive a reduced lump sum and the remainder in the form of an annual income guaranteed for life. Some of the benefits are that the income is guaranteed to last for life, it is index-linked and it is designed specifically to pay for all personal needs. No income tax is payable.

What happens when the damages are awarded

Damages will be paid tax free. However if the sum of money is substantial you should seek expert advice with regard to investment, as you normally have to pay tax on the income from your investment. Sometimes it is desirable to set up a private trust, and your solicitor should advise you on this. This entails putting money or property into the charge of appointed trustee or trustees. Many trusts exist under which the trustee has a wide discretion to use the income of the property to benefit the disabled person, providing extra comforts such as holidays or special equipment.

DRIVING AFTER HEAD INJURY

Many people who have had a head injury are eager to return to driving as soon as possible. However there are certain legal considerations and sensible precautions that have to be observed, because driving a car is a very complex skill with potentially lethal consequences.

Legally, if you have had an injury which affects your fitness to drive, and the effects of that injury are likely to last for three months or more, you must inform the Medical Advisory Branch of the Driving Vehicle Licensing Centre (DVLC). In practice any head injury which involves staying in hospital for more than two–three days may impair your driving ability and you should therefore inform the DVLC and your insurance company. The DVLC will then write to your GP or hospital consultant, who will then give an opinion about your abilities. The final decision rests with the DVLC. If you have had an epileptic seizure, you will not be eligible for a driving licence until you have gone a full two years without a seizure. In some cases, if there is a very high risk of epileptic seizures, a licence may not be granted.

There are a number of subtle, hidden problems which may adversely affect your ability to drive. These could include poor concentration, slowed reactions, perceptual problems (difficulties with interpreting what you see), visual difficulties (double or blurred vision), memory problems and inability to control temper. It is a sensible precaution to have a full expert assessment at a disabled driving centre. There are a number scattered around the UK (for example, Banstead Mobility Centre, Park Road, Banstead, Surrey, SM7 3EE). Some centres offer a multidisciplinary assessment and the option to drive a specially adapted car. These centres are also very helpful in giving advice on modification to cars, if a particular physical disability makes this necessary.

An Ideal Head Injury Service

In the UK, current service provision for people with head injury is sharply concentrated on intensive care and, if you are lucky, on acute care up to about six months after injury. However, when the immediate emergency is over, there is little in the way of rehabilitation or retraining to help the individual return to an independent or productive life. Neuropsychological rehabilitation in specialist units has been shown to be effective in helping individuals to become more independent. Because of limited finances to fund placement at these units, patients are often discharged into the care of relatives, sadly with little help or advice. The number of specialist brain injury rehabilitation units is small in the UK compared with, for example, the USA, Australia and Israel. In those countries the insurance companies will fund rehabilitation so that the person with the head injury has the chance to return to the highest level of independence, which means that, ultimately, the final settlement will be smaller. Rehabilitation makes financial sense for the insurance companies.

Services for head-injured people are generally inadequate because the authorities' allocation of resources to this area has not kept up with increasing demand and because services for head-injured people have a low priority on most budgets. One can fancifully visualize an ideal service which would have a number of components relating to the various stages of head injury.

The first stage of head injury is that of the initial trauma. As stated in Chapter 2, if there is a medical emergency this is usually well covered by intensive care facilities and greatly improved medical technology which increases the likelihood of the patient's life being saved. However, at this stage, the provision of information and support for family members is of vital importance, but is often overlooked amidst the technology. Also, if the injury is mild or moderate, there is a strong possibility that the patient will slip through the net and be discharged with no adequate information or advice, only to experience severe physical, mental and emotional difficulties later. If some form of information or brief follow-up counselling service could be provided, it would certainly help.

The second stage involves acute rehabilitation, either as an in-patient or as an out-patient. Good local services are few and far between. An ideal model would have a district rehabilitation team which would contain a mix of professionals interested in and knowledgeable about head injury (doctor, clinical psychologist, occupational therapist, speech therapist, physiotherapist, social worker, Headway co-ordinator). This would mean that more emphasis could be given to the cognitive and emotional/behavioural deficits rather than solely focusing on the physical and medical aspects of rehabilitation. This team would act as a resource to link up with the acute stage and long-term care needs of patients.

A third stage of service provision involves community integration. This would include vocational rehabilitation, access to job opportunities, sheltered employment and a place of dignity for those who cannot work, as provided by a Headway House (a day centre for people with head injury). A range of residential options would also be needed for those not living with their family. These options might include high dependency units for people who require full-time nursing care; medium dependency four–six bedded units in the community run as group homes, with staff support and monitoring; and low dependency flats or units, for individuals to live independently with a minimum level of supervision from a professional or warden who is employed to 'keep an eye' on residents. The overriding aim of these three different levels of residential accommodation is to encourage independence and prevent institutionalization. People with a head injury would be actively involved in the planning and running of these homes, and these homes would provide long-term accommodation in a normal environment: that is, a house in the community. A further aspect of long-term care is the provision of opportunities for respite care, as in reality the burden of care normally falls squarely on the shoulders of the families. This assistance in terms of respite care, or holiday relief, is vital if families are to continue to carry the burden of care without unacceptable levels of stress.

In the USA, and to a lesser extent in the UK, the case management system has evolved. A case manager takes responsibility for the management of individual patient care and ensures that a co-ordinated approach ensues through all the different stages of care, from the acute services to long-term community integration. The case manager is like a clinical co-ordinator, requisitioning different therapists and organizing treatment when and where they are needed. Having one key person addressing all the needs of the patient offers much-needed continuity. The case manager needs to have extensive knowledge of the problems and of the needs of the person with the head injury and the family.

LETTING GO: LONG-TERM ADJUSTMENT

There comes a point on the long road of rehabilitation when family, carers and the person with the head injury have to accept that life after head injury will not be the same. Recovery can take many years and may never be complete. This does not mean saying, "This is it, this is how things are going to be for always", and giving up, but it does mean realizing the change, and accepting that the old life before the accident is over. The person with the head injury is not going to be a brilliant lawyer, a great dancer or a marathon runner. That life, with those goals and aspirations, is past. But just as that life has ended, a new life with fresh goals and unknown horizons starts.

One brave individual who had a head injury acknowledged with painful honesty, "What I was, I am not. What I was, I am never going to be again." This acceptance leads to new beginnings, the struggle to redefine and develop a new sense of self. This is enormously difficult; it is much easier to go on wanting to be the same as the old person before the accident. People develop a 'self-image' over the course of their lives. If you have had a particular self-image for 25 years, it is not going to change overnight just because you have been in an accident and your brain has been shaken around. The same is true for parents and friends. For a person to accept that their loved one, who looks the same, has the same hair, eyes, nose and smile, is no longer the same, is enormously difficult. This letting go of the old and embracing the new is part of the real work of rehabilitation.

It is essential to be flexible enough to accept that things have changed. Things are different — not good, not bad, but different. Family life is different for parents who thought their son had flown the nest and now see an adult return as a dependent child. Married life is different for the wife who has to step into her husband's shoes and take on new responsibilities. For the person with the head injury, expectations have to be altered as regards work life; the challenge is no longer 'how to get to the top', but 'how to occupy yourself meaningfully and feel useful'. Also expectations have to be changed as regards social life because, inevitably, old friends are lost with the demise of an old lifestyle and new friends will be made. Every cloud has a silver lining. Family, friends and professional carers need to help the person with the injury feel good about themselves because of the things they can do — not bad because of the things they cannot do.

One positive way of viewing this process is to see it as a 'second chance'. The person did not die, he is still there, and now you have a second chance, at a life which is essentially different. Courage, strength, support and advice can come from meeting and sharing with people who have been through, or are going through, a similar situation. The network of small self-help and support groups can be a vital life-line in coping. It is comforting to know that you are not alone, and that others have shared the same problems and felt the same despair. Headway National Head Injuries Association has developed enormously over the last decade. If there is not a branch near where you live, why not start one up, as there are many others out there who would want to meet you. Many local branches were formed by parents and relatives burning with frustration, desperate to share and in need of a means to funnel energy and anger.

Finding New Meaning: Matthew's Story

"I used to be a very successful accountant. I was top of my class at school, obtained a 'first' at university and was aiming to achieve all the world could offer. My goal in life was to outdo everybody else, to be the most intelligent, attractive and successful in everything. My accident left me very disabled. I still pushed myself through rehabilitation, being the physiotherapist's star pupil. At the end of formal rehabilitation my achievements plateaued off. I began to realize that I'd never get back to what I was or achieve any of my worldly ambitions. The neuro-psychologist, who carried out some tests on me, said that my intellectual abilities were now in the average range, whereas before I'd been in the superior range — the top 5 per cent. I went through a really bad patch where I was angry, bitter and frustrated: 'Why me?' I could literally have killed the person driving the other car. I started to drink too much. I was aggressive and abusive to my wife, who had been marvellous and had really stood by me through thick and thin. Our marriage was teetering on the edge of the cliff.

I started seeing a counsellor who helped me to come to terms with some of the changes. A year later, my wife and I decided to have a child. Our daughter is now three years old and I love her very much — she makes me so happy. We have another one on the way which we are all looking forward to. It is eight years since my accident and I can honestly say that I am a happy man nowadays. I realize I have changed my goals in life. The most important goal for me has become that of enriching my relationships, especially with my wife, children and friends. I am also learning how important it is to be able to play and have fun, rather than always striving to achieve. I have learned to appreciate the moment rather than constantly aiming to be somewhere else. I carry out some work which involves making and selling clay pots and vases. This might not seem like much, but the actual act of creating gives me a great deal of satisfaction. I also do some voluntary driving and I'm involved with a local charity. We do not have much money. I see people racing past me, caught up in the rat race, and I sometimes think, 'That could have been me', but I do not envy them. The accident changed my life, turned my values upside down and has changed me as a person — probably for the better." ■

I hope that at the end of this book, if you are a person with a head injury, or a relative of a head-injured person, you have gained something — whether it be practical advice, reassurance or just identifying with the stories of others in a similar, difficult situation. If you are a professional, I hope the doors of understanding and insight have been opened slightly and that you will have greater knowledge and understanding to offer to anyone affected by head injury. All of these insights into the subject of head injury must help in the difficult process of adjusting and letting go of the old life and rebuilding a fruitful and fulfilling new life.

PREVENTION OF HEAD INJURY

You can't change the past, but you can help prevent head injuries to yourself and others in the future.

Wear a safety belt

Every time you drive or ride in a car, insist that everyone wears one. *Never* drink and drive. Air bags also increase safety.

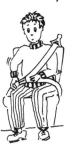

Be careful around your home

Use care with ladders and on stairs. Watch out for other hazards, such as open cabinet doors overhead.

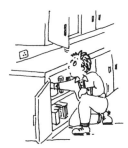

Wear a helmet

Whenever you're on a motorcycle, bicycle or horse, or if you play any sport that involves a high risk of head injury, wear a helmet.

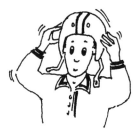

Watch children carefully

Be especially careful when they're in highchairs, strollers or places where they could fall. Use restraining belts whenever possible.

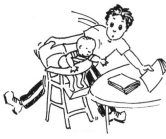

Never shake a child

Shaking anyone can cause brain damage.

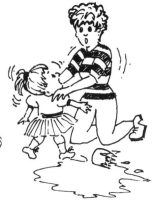

Don't dive into unfamiliar water

Always know how deep water is before you dive or slide.

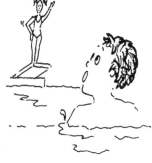

Glossary

Understanding Medical and Technical Terms

ACALCULIA   Inability to perform simple problems of arithmetic.

ACUITY   Sharpness or quality of sensation.

AGEUSIA   Partial or total loss of the sense of taste.

AGNOSIA   Failure to recognize familiar objects and know the meaning or significance of things.

AGRAPHIA   Loss of the ability to write.

AMBLYOPI   Blindness.

AMNESIA   Partial or total loss of the ability to remember things which have been done or experienced. (See post-traumatic amnesia and retrograde amnesia.)

ANEURISM   A balloon-like deformity in the wall of a blood vessel — may eventually burst, causing haemorrhage.

ANOSMI   Failure to smell.

ANOXIA   Lack of oxygen supply to brain cells.

ANTICONVULSANT   Medication used to decrease the possibility of a seizure (eg. Dilantin, Phenobarbital, Mysoline, Tegretol).

APHASIA   Reduction of the ability to communicate with others through the use of language. Receptive aphasia is not understanding the language of others. Expressive aphasia is a reduction in the ability to use language, for example naming and making mistakes in word usage.

APRAXIA   Inability to plan and perform purposeful movements, while still having the ability to move and be aware of the movement.

ATAXIA   Unsteadiness of movement; muscular unco-ordination when voluntary movements are attempted.

BEHAVIOUR MODIFICATION   A form of therapy using the principle of learning, aimed at changing behaviour by altering the rewards and consequences of that behaviour.

BRAIN PLASTICITY   The ability of intact brain cells to take over functions of damaged cells; plasticity diminishes as we get older.

BRAIN STEM/ MID-BRAIN   A bundle of nerve tissues below the main hemisphere at the top of the spinal cord. Controls bodily functions such as consciousness, wakefulness and breathing.

BURR HOLE   A hole drilled in the skull.

CEREBELLUM   A lump of tissue behind the brain stem regulating fine motor movements.

CEREBRAL HEMISPHERES   The two side-by-side halves of the cerebrum.

CEREBROSPINAL FLUID (CSF)   The clear, colourless fluid in the spaces inside and around the brain and the spinal cord.

CEREBRUM   The large walnut-like part of the brain, divided into two hemispheres (right and left) and different areas called lobes (frontal, temporal, parietal, occipital).

CIRCUMLOCUTION Use of other words to describe a specific word or idea which cannot be remembered; not getting to the point.

CLONUS Rapidly alternating involuntary contraction and relaxation of a muscle in response to a sudden stretch.

CLOSED HEAD INJURY Damage to the brain where there is no penetration from the scalp or skull through to brain tissue. Often there is no injury to scalp or skull.

COGNITIVE ABILITIES Mental abilities such as thinking, remembering, planning, understanding, concentrating and using language.

COMA State of unconsciousness, the depth of which can be measured by the Glasgow Coma Scale, allowing a grading of coma by observation of eye opening, limb movements and speech.

CONCRETE THINKING A style of thinking in which the individual sees each situation as unique and is unable to generalize from the similarities between situations.

CONCUSSION Unconsciousness after a blow to the head.

CONFABULATION Verbalizations about people, places or events with no basis in reality.

CONTRACTURE Joints and muscles that are not used regularly, quickly become stiff, rendering them resistant to stretching. Eventually the joints become fixed, restricting movement, and can be released only by surgery.

CONTRALATERAL   Opposite side.

CONTRECOUP   Bruising of brain tissue on the opposite side to where
                       the blow was struck.

CONTUSION   A bruise caused by a blow with a blunt object.

CRANIOTOM   Operation to open the skull. Usually involves cutting a
                       trap-door in the bone of the skull exactly over the blood
                       clot and then washing the clot away. The bone is then
                       put back into place and heals firmly, usually after three
                       to four weeks.

CRANIUM   The bony skull. (Intracranial — inside the skull.)

CT SCAN   Computerized Axial Tomography (CAT for short). A
                       large doughnut-shaped machine which is actually an x-
                       ray camera that can take pictures of a person's brain in
                       slices. Because it is able, photographically, to 'peel
                       away' layers of tissue, it can pinpoint problem areas,
                       especially bruises and blood accumulation, and can
                       help to determine if surgery is needed.

DEMENTIA   Generally impaired thinking, damaged intellectual
                       functioning.

DIFFUSE AXONAL   Widespread tearing of nerve fibres across the whole of
INJURY (DAI)   the brain.

DIPLOPIA   Double vision.

DISINHIBITION   Difficulty in controlling urges and impulses to speak, act
                       or show emotion.

DURA MATER	The outermost of the three membranes covering the brain.
DYSARTHRIA	Difficulty with articulation and pronunciation of words, due to slowness, weakness or unco-ordination of tone of muscles.
DYSLEXIA	Difficulty in reading and spelling.
DYSPHAGIA	Difficulty in swallowing.
DYSPHASIA	(Same as Aphasia)
DYSPRAXIA	(Same as Apraxia)
EDEMA	Swelling of the brain.
EEG (ELECTRO-ENCEPHALOGRAM)	Electrodes attached to the scalp measure the electrical activity (waves) in the brain and show the results, either on graph paper or a screen. If someone has a moderate or severe head injury, it is likely to show an abnormal brain wave pattern or an irregular brain wave speed.
EMBOLISM	Sudden blockage of an artery by a clot.
EMOTIONAL LABILITY	Rapid and drastic changes in emotional state (laughing, crying, anger) that are inappropriate.
EXECUTIVE FUNCTIONS	Planning, organizing, problem solving, sequencing, prioritizing, self-monitoring, self-correcting, controlling or altering behaviour and judgement.
EXTRADURAL	Between the dura and the skull.

FLACCID	Floppy, without tone; limp.
FRONTAL LOBE	The part of each cerebral hemisphere primarily concerned with planning and organizing, attention and the control and regulation of behaviour and emotion.
FRUSTRATION TOLERANCE	The ability to persist in completing a task despite apparent difficulty.
GASTROSTOMY	The creation of an opening into the stomach for the administration of foods and fluids when swallowing is impossible.
GLASGOW COMA SCALE	A numerical score given to head-injured patients, starting immediately after injury, to measure degree of unconsciousness. A score of seven or less indicates that the person is in a coma. A maximum score of 15 indicates that the person can speak coherently, obey commands to move, and can spontaneously open his eyes.
HAEMATOMA	Blood clot. When the brain is bruised it may bleed. The collection of this blood into 'pools' or 'clots' is known as haematoma. When the pool of blood actually forms within the brain, it is known as an 'intracerebral haematoma'. When the blood collects between the brain and the dura membrane, it is called a 'subdural haematoma'. These clots of blood press against the brain tissue, causing damage.
HAEMORRHAGE	Blood loss; bleeding.
HEMIANOPIA	Loss of one side of the field of vision.

HEMIPLEGIA	Loss of power in one side of the body.
HYDROCEPHALUS	Accumulation of cerebrospinal fluid within the brain, sometimes at high pressure, causing expansion of the ventricles and possible injury to the brain.
HYPOTHALAMUS	A nerve centre deep in the diencephalon area which controls the autonomic nervous system, food intake, sexual rhythms, emotions and memory.
HYPOXIA	Diminished availability of oxygen to body tissues.
INFARCT	An area where brain cells have died as a result of loss of blood supply.
INTENSIVE CARE	An area of the hospital where the patient is monitored very carefully by connecting him via tubes and wires to several machines. The activity of the heart shows continually on an electrocardiogram. Blood pressure is recorded by attaching a fine tube to a small artery in the ankle or arm. Pressure inside the skull is measured with a lead from inside the skull. A drip transfusion is put into a vein in the arm, carrying food and fluids. A mechanical ventilator controls breathing.
INTRACRANIAL PRESSURE (ICP)	The pressure inside the skull.
INTRAVENOUS	Tubing inserted into a vein through which fluids and medication can be given.
LIMBIC SYSTEM	A group of deep cortical structures connected to the hypothalamus, governing memory, emotions and basic drives, including sex drive.

MRI (MAGNETIC RESONANCE IMAGING)	The latest diagnostic device combines computer technology and physics. The MRI uses radio frequency and a magnet to chart electrical charges created in the brain. It then converts them into computerized, highly detailed pictures of the brain. MRIs can display both specific and general nerve damage.
MUSCLE TONE	The muscle's readiness to contract or the degree of resistance to movement in a limb or group of muscles. Muscle tone can be normal, increased or decreased.
NASOGASTRIC TUBE	A very fine tube passed down through the nose and throat into the stomach for giving liquid food and pureed meals. Used if there are swallowing difficulties.
NEOLOGISM	Nonsense or made-up word.
NEURON	A nerve cell.
NEURO-TRANSMITTERS	Chemicals made in the nervous system that serve as messengers throughout the nervous system, aiding or interfering with the function of nerve cells.
NYSTAGMUS	Jerking of the eyes, usually following damage to the brain stem.
OCCIPITAL LOBE	The part of each cerebral hemisphere primarily concerned with perception and interpretation of visual information.
OEDEMA	Excess fluid in tissues, causing swelling.
OPEN HEAD INJURY	An injury where there is a penetration of the scalp and skull through to brain tissue.

PARALYSIS	Loss of ability of muscles to contract.
PARAPLEGIA	Paralysis of the lower extremities only. More likely to result from damage to the spinal cord than from a head injury.
PARIETAL LOBE	The part of each cerebral hemisphere primarily concerned with the perception and interpretation of sensation and movement.
PERCEPTION	The ability to make sense out of what one sees, hears, feels, tastes or smells.
PERSEVERATION	Involuntary prolonged repetition of words or actions.
PERSISTENT VEGETATIVE STATE	A long-standing condition in which the patient utters no words and does not follow commands or make any response that is meaningful.
PHOTOPHOBIA	Abnormal sensitivity of the eyes to light.
POST-CONCUSSION SYNDROME	A group of symptoms occurring after mild head injury that may persist for days, weeks or months.
POST-TRAUMATIC AMNESIA (PTA)	Inability to remember continuous events, after a blow to the head which causes an alteration of consciousness, even when the patient is apparently awake.
PROGNOSIS	The outlook for improvement or lack of it.
PSYCHOMETRIC TESTS	Standardized tests which measure mental functioning.

REHABILITATION An active process by which a disabled person realizes his optimal physical, mental and social potential.

RETROGRADE
AMNESIA
Inability to remember events that happened for a period before a blow to the head.

SUBDURAL Between the dura membrane and the brain.

SHUNT (Ventriculovenous shunt.) A device to remove excess fluid or divert blood. Basically it is a U-shaped piece of plastic tube with a valve, which opens at pressure, which can be inserted between an artery and a vein, bypassing the capillary network.

SPASTIC Having stiffness or weakness of the limbs, from loss of higher nervous functioning.

SPINAL CORD The extension of the central nervous system from the brain-stem lodged within the spine; contains long neural pathways to and from the brain.

SUPPOSITORY Medicine contained in a capsule which is inserted into the rectum so that it can be absorbed into the bloodstream.

TEMPORAL LOBE The part of each cerebral hemisphere concerned with sound and language interpretation, and important in memory function.

TRACHEOTOMY A small operation, usually with local anaesthetic, carried out if there is an obstruction of the airways. The windpipe is opened through an incision in the neck just below the Adam's apple, and a plastic tube threaded in to facilitate the passage of air and the evacuation of secretions.

TRANSFER PROGRAMME	Moving one's body between wheelchair and bed, toilet, mat or car without the assistance of another person.
TRAUMA	Damage to any part of the body.
TRAUMATIC BRAIN INJURY	Damage to the brain and/or brain stem due to mechanical injury. Most frequent causes are vehicle accidents, followed by domestic and industrial accidents, sports injuries and assaults.
TREMOR	Regular repetitive movements which may be worse either at rest or on attempted movement.
UNILATERAL	Pertaining to only one side.
VENTILATOR	Also called a respirator. A machine which pumps oxygen-enriched air into the lungs when they are not working efficiently. This encourages quiet breathing and the prevention of coughing and straining, gives the right amount of carbon dioxide to the blood and creates the best conditions for healing the brain.
VENTRICLE	A fluid-filled cavity in the brain.
VESTIBULAR	System in the middle ear which senses movement. Injury can lead to dizziness.
X-RAY	Ordinary X-rays show the bone of the skull. They are useful for ascertaining whether there has been a fracture to the skull, or whether any fragments of bone have been pushed into the brain.

Useful Addresses

Great Britain

Headway National Head Injuries
Association
7 King Edward Court
King Edward Street
Nottingham NG1 lEW
Tel: 01602 240800

Australia

The Head Injury Council of
Australia (HICOA)
PO Box 304
Port Melbourne 3207
Australia 03 696-1388

Canada

Ontario Head Injury Association
PO Box 2388 'Sth B'
St Catherines
Ontario
Canada L2M 7MF

New Zealand

The Head Injured Society (Inc)
Auckland
PO Box 15309
New Lynn
Auckland 7

South Africa

Headway
National Head Injuries Association
PO Box 64310
Highlands North
Johannesburg
2037
Republic of South Africa

USA

National Head Injury Foundation
1776 Massachusetts Ave
N.W. Suit 100
Washington DC 20036

● For details of your local group,
contact the national organization
address above.

Suggestions for Further Reading

For Families and Carers

Gronwall D, Wrightson P & Waddell P, *Head Injury: The Facts,* Oxford University Press, Oxford, 1990.

Senelick R & Ryan C, *Living with Head Injury,* Bantam Premium Books, Washington, 1991.

All booklets published by Headway National Head Injuries Association.

For Professionals

Brooks N (ed), *Closed Head Injury: Psychological, Social and Family Consequences,* Oxford University Press, Oxford, 1984.

Kreutzer J & Wehman P, *Community Integration Following Traumatic Brain Injury,* Paul H Brookes, London, 1990.

Levin H, Eisenberg H & Benton A, *Mild Head Injury,* Oxford University Press, New York/Oxford, 1989.

Muir Giles G & Clark Wilson J, *Brain Injury Rehabilitation,* Chapman-Hall, London, 1993.

Royal College of Physicians Committee on the Young Physically Disabled Report, *Journal of the Royal College of the Physicians of London* 20, pp 160-94, 1986.

Williams J & Kay T, *Head Injury: A Family Matter,* Paul H Brookes, London, 1991.

Wilson B & Moffat N, *Clinical Management of Memory Problems,* Croom Helm, London, 1984.

INDEX